Cocaine Solutions:
Help for Cocaine Abusers
and Their Families

The Haworth Series in Addictions Treatment

Series Editor: F. Bruce Carruth

Cocaine Solutions:
Help for Cocaine Abusers
and Their Families

Jennifer Rice-Licare
Katharine Delaney-McLoughlin

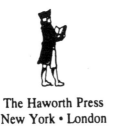

The Haworth Press
New York • London

Cocaine Solutions: Help for Cocaine Abusers and Their Families is Volume Number 4 in the Haworth Series in Addictions Treatment.

The Haworth Press, Inc., 10 Alice Street, Binghamton, NY 13904-1580
EUROSPAN/Haworth, 3 Henrietta Street, London WC2E 8LU England

Library of Congress Cataloging-in-Publication Data

Rice-Licare, Jennifer.
    Cocaine solutions : help for cocaine abusers and their families / Jennifer Rice-Licare, Katharine Delaney-McLoughlin.
        p.   cm. — (Haworth series in addictions treatment ; v. 4)
    Published simultaneously by Harrington Park Press with the same title.
    Includes bibliographical references.
    Inlcudes index.
    ISBN 1-56024-035-0
    1. Cocaine habit — Treatment. 2. Family psychotherapy. I. McLoughlin, Katharine Delaney. II. Title. III. Series.
    [DNLM: 1. Cocaine. 2. Family. 3. Substance Dependence — rehabilitation. WM 280 R497c]
RC568.C6R53 1990b
362.29'88 — dc20
DNLM/DLC
for Library of Congress   90-4843
                                                                                               CIP

CONTENTS

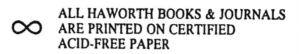

ABOUT THE AUTHORS

Jennifer Rice-Licare, CAC, CAS, CEAP, is a community outreach and education representative for the Seafield Alcoholism Treatment Center in Westhampton Beach, New York. Active in the field of addiction for eight years, she has been a credentialled alcoholism counselor for four years and a certified employee assistance professional for three years. She has been associated with the Smither's Treatment Center in New York, and has worked for Dr. Arnold Washton, a nationally known cocaine authority, and for the Mediplex Substance Abuse Treatment Centers. Ms. Rice-Licare is a prominent speaker on substance abuse and has appeared on several national television programs, including *The Oprah Winfrey Show* and *The Phil Donahue Show*. She is a frequent lecturer at conventions, schools and corporations across the country.

Katharine Delaney-McLoughlin, MA, an experienced cocaine addiction therapist who h as been involved in the field for more tha 10 years, currently works as a freelance consultant. She has worked in several settings including an outpatient clinic, a psychiatric hospital, and a private counseling agency. She has counselled cocaine addicts and their families, alcoholics, and adult children of alcoholics. Ms. Delaney-McLoughlin has a master's degree in forensic psychology from the City University of New York John Jay College of Criminal Justice. She has also received extensive training in chemical dependency counseling. She has spoken at conferences and seminars for both the public and professionals on cocaine addiction.

Foreword

No other drug has caught people's attention as cocaine has done today. Barely a decade ago, it was a "benign" drug, fashionable and expensive, the jet-setter's most sought after chemical, the stuff that gave a new meaning to weekend parties and resort vacations. As the number of addicted people grew and as the Emergency Room visits increased, some of the gloss and charm of cocaine began to wane. The drug, however, did not vanish from the scene. A perverse enterpreneurial system modified it, pre-packaged it and sold it actually cheaper, thus making it available to the young and less affluent sections of the society. Crack has turned our world upside down, putting money into the hands of teenagers, giving them far more wealth and power than their parents ever had. This enormously addictive form of cocaine has caused our jail cells to swell to a bursting point while straining an already overburdened mental health system to its limits.

About 12 million people use cocaine in the U.S. in any given year. According to data published by the National Institute on Drug Abuse, there were less than 5,000 Emergency Room visits in the year 1982-1983 as a direct result of using cocaine. By 1986-1987, however, the number of visits had soared to 25,000. Despite intensive efforts to stop the drug from entering the country, our borders seem ever more porous where cocaine is concerned. Most experts now agree that, if the cocaine epidemic has to be contained and eventually eradicated, efforts need to be directed at the user — that is to say that those who are already victims of cocaine, need treatment, and those who are vulnerable to the drug, prevented from becoming new users.

It is, therefore, especially gratifying to welcome the book by Jennifer Rice-Licare and Katherine Delaney-McLoughlin. The authors have written a clear, no-nonsense book on cocaine, devoid of jargon and excessive medical details, suitable not only for those who are already in the throes of addiction and desperately seeking a way out, but also for family members who may be concerned for their spouses or children. The book is generously sprinkled with true lift stories that help to bring the various aspects of the disease into sharper focus. That the non-addicted family members also need support and counselling is addressed in the chapter "The Family." I hope the readers find this book as helpful and interesting as I have.

Premkumar Peter, MD
Clinical Assistant Professor of Psychiatry
New York Medical College
Valhalla, NY

Preface

When I was asked to write the Preface for *Cocaine Solutions* I — a recovering cocaine addict — was a bit skeptical as to what the material would say. As I read through the book looking for something wrong, I found something right. This book really spoke to me because it covers everything anyone needs to know about cocaine addiction, and more important, living in recovery.

I've been clean and sober from cocaine, alcohol, and all mind-altering chemicals since November 8, 1983. As I've continued to grow in my recovery and profession, my eyes and ears have seen and heard things that have set me free. This book continues to do so. I'm free because during my recovery I've been green and growing rather than ripe and rotten.

This book doesn't miss anything or anyone. It has cocaine addicts, alcoholics, sex abuse survivors, co-dependents, and sex addicts sharing their stories. It doesn't get any better than this! Sharing those powerful secrets takes all the power out of them.

I believe that to be recovering is pure freedom. I also believe we have to prove it everyday. If we don't, we relapse. Recovery for me also means we forgive ourselves. When we forgive ourselves and ask others to forgive us, they must, even if they don't love us anymore.

This book should be read by everyone who can read. If they can't read, someone should read it to them. Cocaine is killing a whole generation. That generation is the "now" generation. Our government and all people should know that this ain't no Black drug problem, no Colombian drug problem, no Mexican drug problem, or no poor white folk drug problem. This cocaine problem is everyone's problem — all colors, creeds, and religions. Until we realize and acknowledge that, the problem will only grow because cocaine is everywhere.

Our nations has a war on drugs that isn't working. I agree partially with interdiction, and I agree totally with punishment and with education as the best deterrent to our war on drugs. But until there is treatment on demand in America for each and every citizen, the war on drugs will never be more than a political toy.

The authors' efforts are appreciated by this cocaine addict who now happens to be clean and sober.

Thomas "Hollywood" Henderson
Former NFL Linebacker
Lecturer; National Consultant
Sierra Tucson Treatment Center
Tucson, AZ

Acknowledgements

We would like to acknowledge Lisa Stolley for her invaluable editorial assistance. We would also like to recognize the following people who contributed to the chapter on adolescence: Wendy H. Bausch-Davenson, Steven DeMartino, Rosemary Rowley, James Rowley, Karen Glass-Saraga and Patricia Rose Attia.

We appreciate the help provided by the Seafield Center, Barbara Eisenstat, Katherine Janis McLoughlin and Anne Lyons. We are also very thankful to Thomas Henderson and Dr. Prem Peter for writing the Preface and the Foreword, and for the wonderful help and insight they each provided.

We are extremely grateful to our husbands, Tom Licare and John McLoughlin, whose support helped us to write the book.

Chapter 1

Prologue

This book is designed for anyone who is interested in the use and abuse of cocaine.

We, the authors, especially want to reach those of you who are concerned that a loved one may be addicted to cocaine: maybe your daughter has not been acting in her usual manner, or you are concerned because your husband has cashed his paycheck and there is less money for household expenses; perhaps your friend goes into unexplained rages, or you know that something is wrong with your own life and it may have begun with snorting cocaine.

Oddly enough, although the newspaper and magazine headlines are trumpeting the rise of cocaine use, the public receives very little information about the cocaine problem. Indeed, some believe that it is merely another fad, a lot of media attention on not much of anything. Others believe that cocaine addiction is the same as other addictions — alcohol, amphetamines, tranquilizers, etc. — and should be treated no differently.

This debate is academic for cocaine addicts and for those who know them. It is the addicts' family and friends who watch their loved ones travel the road to self-destruction. Not only are addicts themselves destroyed, but entire families pay the price, financially, emotionally and mentally.

A distinguishing mark of cocaine addiction is its expense. Since cocaine costs a lot of money, stealing is frequently a sign of cocaine addiction. The financial price, however, is the least of the consequences of the use and abuse of cocaine. Families suffer because the addict no longer loves them, but loves the drug, causing harm that can last a lifetime.

It is frightening to think that someone you know and love could be "one of them." Parents have a particularly difficult time acknowledging that their teenager or child may be smoking crack. If they don't know it, what can they do to stop him or her from using cocaine? How do they confront the child? How do they avoid believing that they are responsible for their child's addiction?

There is help for addicts and their families. We, the authors, know this because we are recovered drug addicts. Both of us have also seen countless numbers of people recover from cocaine addiction. This book provides information on how the addict and family can get help. There is also some discussion regarding the obstacles to recovery and the ways to overcome them. There are also some life stories of recovered addicts to show an addict's life. Hopefully, you will relate to one of the stories or you may gain a better understanding of those who have been caught in the disease of addiction. Lastly, we have developed a list of cocaine treatment resources where you may seek help.

Part of obtaining help may be participating in one of the Twelve-Step programs, especially Cocaine Anonymous. Twelve-Step programs are expanding and are used in conjunction with most successful cocaine addiction treatment programs. All Twelve-Step programs, including Alcoholics Anonymous, Cocaine Anonymous, Narcotics Anonymous, Al-Anon, Co-Anon and Nar-Anon, are based on the principles originally outlined in the book *Alcoholics Anonymous*. The twelve steps are listed below, reprinted with permission from Alcoholics Anonymous:

1. We admitted we were powerless over alcohol (Cocaine Anonymous substitutes "cocaine and all other mind altering substances"); that our lives had become unmanageable.
2. Came to believe that a Power greater than ourselves could restore us to sanity.
3. Made a decision to turn our will and our lives over to the care of God as we understood Him.
4. Made a searching and fearless moral inventory of ourselves.
5. Admitted to God, to ourselves and to another human being the exact nature of our wrongs.
6. Were entirely ready to have God remove all these defects of character.

7. Humbly asked Him to remove our shortcomings.
8. Made a list of all persons we had harmed, and became willing to make amends to them.
9. Made direct amends to such people wherever possible, except when to do so would injure them or others.
10. Continued to take personal inventory and when we were wrong promptly admitted it.
11. Sought through prayer and meditation to improve our conscious contact with God, as we understood Him, praying only for knowledge of His will for us and the power to carry that out.
12. Having had a spiritual awakening as the result of these steps, we tried to carry this message to alcoholics (addicts) and to practice these principles in all our affairs.

It must be emphasized that no one has real control over another person. We believe in a saying often repeated by people in Alcoholics Anonymous, "you can carry the message, but you can't carry the drunk." All of us can carry the message to the addicts, but we cannot make them stop using cocaine. We can tell them they are able to stop using and here's how, but it is really up to them. They have to want to stop using, and we can't do that for them no matter how hard we try.

Chapter 2

Cocaine and Cocaine Addiction

THE ORIGIN OF COCAINE

Cocaine is derived from the leaves of the coca plants harvested in Central and South America. Cocaine was used centuries ago in its most natural form by the Indians of the region, who chewed it in their religious ceremonies and while working in the mountains.

Cocaine outside Central and South America dates to the middle 1800s when chemists in Europe separated the cocaine alkaloid from the leaves. They discovered that it had two major effects — as an anesthetic and as a stimulant. Initially used to anesthetize the eye during surgery, it was soon applied to other parts of the body as well. But its effect as a stimulant was what made cocaine popular for nonmedicinal uses. Sigmund Freud experimented with cocaine by inhaling (snorting) it through his nose. He initially wrote glowing reports about its effects, saying that it increased self-confidence and alertness and enabled him to work through the night. He changed his views after medical case studies indicated that the drug was addicting.

Cocaine was first exported legally to the United States. In fact, the beverage Coca-Cola® originally contained cocaine. In the early twentieth century, however, those ingredients were removed from the drink when Congress enacted the Harrison Act outlawing cocaine and a number of other drugs.

Beginning in the 1960s, cocaine became known as the "Champagne of Drugs" for its popularity among the jetsetters. Its high price made it a preserve of the wealthy, but the drug became more widespread as its cost came down. It was regarded as safe and nonaddictive and it became fashionable in some circles to provide cocaine at parties. By the 1970s, cocaine had become popular among a wide range of people.

The assumption that cocaine is not addictive, i.e., that it is not "destructive" like other drugs, has probably contributed highly to the ease with which people have been caught up by cocaine addiction. Public attention was drawn to its danger in 1986 when two well-known athletes — Len Bias, a basketball star at the University of Maryland, and Don Rogers, defensive back of the Cleveland Browns — died from cardiac arrest caused by cocaine use.

Since then, stories about the famous and their cocaine addictions have been reported in the media on an almost daily basis. The most frightening aspect of cocaine, however, is the spread of its most addictive form, freebase cocaine. The introduction of crack as pre-packaged freebase cocaine in 1985 has transformed cocaine use. Relatively cheap, crack is now used by poorer and younger people who previously may not have used cocaine.

This has serious repercussions for American society. First, poorer people are more likely to steal in order to support a crack/ cocaine habit. Second, adolescents may be more vulnerable than adults to possible physical problems, including brain damage, because their body systems have not fully matured.

Finally, since crack is so highly addictive, the drug makes it far more likely for casual experimenters to become "hooked."

BIOCHEMICAL EFFECTS OF COCAINE USE

Cocaine's use as an anesthetic is due to its vasoconstrictor effect. It slows down the flow of blood throughout the circulatory system which makes it useful as an anesthetic during surgery, as well as directly affecting the heart and circulatory system by raising the blood pressure and increasing the respiratory rate.

All drugs affect the central nervous system, but they do so in different ways; these different effects are used to classify the drugs. There are four major classifications of psychoactive drugs: sedatives (alcohol, tranquilizers); opioids (morphine, heroin, etc.); hallucinogens (marijuana, LSD, PCP, STP, etc.); and stimulants, which include amphetamines and cocaine. As a stimulant, cocaine affects the body—regardless of how it is used—in the following ways:

- increased heart rate
- increased pulse rate
- increased blood pressure
- loss of appetite
- sleeplessness/insomnia
- alertness
- dilated pupils

While cocaine is a stimulant, its effects differ markedly from other stimulants. Cocaine use is characterized by "crashing" and "bingeing." Cocaine's initial effect is one that can be described as a euphoric feeling which lasts only a short while (a couple of hours at the most when snorted, and half an hour at most when smoked). When the euphoria ends, the user experiences "letdown," and depression, and wants to regain that initial good feeling. The result is a vicious cycle:

cocaine intake —-> euphoric feeling —-> crash —-> craving for cocaine —-> cocaine intake —-> a feeling of lesser euphoria —-> bigger crash —-> more cocaine —-> . . .

This process goes on until the user cannot physically continue or the money runs out. This is the "bingeing"—using cocaine until it is gone (up to a few days and nights), resting for a few days until the body and finances are ready again, using cocaine again, etc.

Cocaine's addictive properties are dramatically demonstrated by animal experiments. In experiments where rats obtain cocaine by pressing a lever, rats would take cocaine until they died (Holzman). In experiments with monkeys, monkeys self-administered the cocaine and demonstrated cocaine-abuse behaviors such as hyperactivity, paranoid psychosis, self-mutilation, convulsions, cardiovascular collapse and respiratory failure (Holzman).

The cycle of bingeing and craving probably has a physiological basis. Scientists believe they have established the chemical basis for the initial cycle of euphoria and craving in what they call the dopamine-depletion theory.

The brain is composed of circuits that are themselves composed of hundreds of billions of nerve cells that communicate with one another across gaps known as synapses. Chemicals known as neurotransmitters carry the cells' messages across these gaps. Three of the body's natural neurotransmitters are epinephrine, norepinephrine and dopamine. These chemicals affect the pleasure center of the brain and therefore are responsible for an elevated, positive mood.

The neurotransmitters are sent from one nerve cell to attach themselves to receptors located on the receiving nerve cell. The dopamine-depletion theory asserts that cocaine keeps the nerve cells from receiving dopamine because it attaches itself to the receptor to which the dopamine normally attaches itself; the dopamine remains in the synapse. This means the dopamine continues to discharge its "elevated, positive mood" signals, bringing pleasure to the cocaine user. But the dopamine is then lost from the synapse, preventing its neural signals from reaching the appropriate nerve cells in the pleasure center. At the same time, the receiving nerve cells are thought to become supersensitive to the dopamine in an effort to compensate for its deficit.

Since cocaine interferes with the body's balance of neurotransmitters, the physical effects of withdrawal from cocaine may be the symptoms of the body trying to regain that balance. At Fair Oaks Hospital in New Jersey, an experiment was conducted in which fifty chronic cocaine users were medicated with bromocriptine, a drug that is believed to affect the dopamine receptor sites (Gold). Bromocriptine masked or eliminated cocaine withdrawal's physical effects, indicating that these are symptoms of neurotransmitter depletion.

There are other theories regarding the bingeing and craving cycle. At Columbia-Presbyterian Hospital in New York City, cocaine addicts who were also depressed were treated with an antidepressant, impipramine (Holzman). Impipramine seems to block the cocaine euphoria and reduce the user's craving by acting on neural circuits that contain the neurotransmitters norepinephrine and serotinin. In conjunction with using impipramine, patients are given vitamins that rebuild the neurotransmitters.

One cocaine expert, Dr. Arnold Washton of the Washton Institute in New York, believes that cocaine becomes as crucial to the user as the biological needs for water, food and shelter. Dr. Washton states that cocaine affects the limbic portion of the brain, the storehouse for the primary drives such as thirst and hunger. In doing so, it produces a feeling that the drug is crucial to the user's well-being.

Cocaine's effects depend on a variety of factors. These include: (1) the quality of cocaine; (2) the method by which it is used (this especially affects physical side effects); (3) how often the drug is used; (4) whether it is used with other drugs, including alcohol; and (5) the user's physical and mental health. Environment also plays a role in the use of cocaine—whether the drug is taken at a party, alone, or in a crack house. But the behavioral and psychological effects of cocaine addiction are virtually the same, regardless of the method of use.

COCAINE EFFECTS ON THE USER

Cocaine affects users in a variety of ways. Their mood can swing from joyous to enraged, loving to hateful, passive to violent. Cocaine users may talk a lot, jiggle one or both legs or restlessly drum their fingers on the table.

Since cocaine use causes dehydration, users may frequently lick their lips or drink a lot of liquids. Cocaine users sometimes grind their teeth, chew their lips or packs of gum. More often than not, the cocaine user will puff away on cigarette after cigarette.

Users have reported that their perceptions change when they use cocaine. Sometimes they experience hallucinations; more often their thinking is distorted. Many cocaine addicts become paranoid; it is not uncommon for them to talk of being chased by the CIA or others who are "out to get them." People who abuse cocaine often lose their appetite and eat little, enough to suffer from vitamin deficiencies. For example, it was found at Fair Oaks Hospital that 73% of the cocaine addict patients suffered from vitamin deficiency, mostly of B-6 (Gold, *The Facts About Drugs and Alcohol*).

Cocaine has a reputation for increasing sexual desire and performance. Beginning users sometimes feel this to be true, but steady, long-term users find just the opposite. With high doses of cocaine, sexual needs and/or desires seem to decrease. In fact, as with any drug used chronically and heavily, cocaine will usually replace sexual activity.

Most importantly, cocaine is not a "safe drug." The National Institute of Drug Abuse has reported that cocaine-related visits to emergency rooms increased from 3,296 in 1981 to 9,946 in 1985. Cocaine, more than other drugs, has dangerous effects on the heart. Regular use of cocaine can cause heart palpitations, angina (severe pain around the heart), arrhythmia (irregular heartbeat) and even a heart attack.

THE COCAINE HIGH

The cocaine high is that initial euphoric feeling that users experience when taking cocaine in any form. The way in which cocaine is taken into the body affects how the user experiences the high. For example, injecting and smoking cocaine will usually produce more immediate and pronounced effects than snorting.

There are five ways in which cocaine is most often used:

1. inhaled intranasally (snorting)
2. injected intravenously (shooting up)
3. smoked/freebase
4. smoked/crack
5. smoked/basuco

1. Inhaled Intranasally (Snorting)

Cocaine is snorted only in the form of cocaine hydrochloride, which is usually in a powder form. This variant of cocaine is derived from the coca base that is extracted from the cocaine sulfate or paste that is processed from the coca leaves.

Cocaine snorters usually snort the cocaine hydrochloride by separating the powder into thin lines on a piece of glass or mirror and inhaling it into the nose through a rolled-up dollar bill. Some snorters like to use a tiny spoon. As an anesthetic, cocaine numbs the mucous membranes immediately; users often rub it on their gums to obtain the numbing sensation. In its powder form, the drug dissolves on the mucous membranes and is absorbed through the capillary walls. It then enters the bloodstream and flows to the brain. The cocaine user feels the effects of the cocaine in approximately three minutes.

A snorter usually buys cocaine in grams or fractions of grams meaning that he or she has to spend more money at the outset than any other cocaine user. One gram usually costs about $75-$100, an ounce (28 grams) about $1,800 to $3,000.

Snorting cocaine has direct impact on the nose, throat and ears. Often the user will experience congestion, sneezing, hoarseness, head colds, throat infections, asthma and bronchitis. The drug, if it remains undissolved, also causes burns and sores. Chronic snorting can cause the mucous linings of the nose to deteriorate; the drug actually eats through the cartilage.

Cocaine is usually only about 40-50% pure since it is cut with one or more adulterants, most commonly mannitol (a relatively safe filler used in the making of pills), caffeine, lactose or sucrose (types of sugar), inosital (vitamin B), amphetamines and quinine. It can also be cut with local anesthetics such as lidocaine, procaine, tetracaine, benzocaine and butacaine. The adulterants can have side effects of their own, such as: depression, ringing in ears, nausea and headaches.

Most people begin their cocaine use by snorting, since that method does not have as negative an image as injecting or smoking the drug.

Cocaine hydrochloride can only be snorted or injected since it evaporates when it is heated.

2. Intravenous Injection (Shooting Up)

Since cocaine hydrochloride dissolves in water, it can be made into a solution and injected by syringe directly into a vein. This effect is more immediate than when cocaine is snorted; only about thirty to sixty seconds are needed for the drug to reach the brain. Fewer people inject cocaine since this method is considered rather sinister: only "addicts" shoot up. Most people who inject cocaine do so in combination with other drugs, more commonly heroin, known as "speedballs."

Injection is the most immediately dangerous way of using cocaine. Side effects include heart attacks, angina and endocarditis. Simply using needles has risks of its own, among them hepatitis, damaged veins, skin abscesses and AIDS. Finally, injection creates the chance of an overdose, often a fatal one.

3. Smoking/Freebase

Of all methods of using cocaine, freebasing — smoking the drug in lumps from a pipe — produces the most powerful and immediate effect. The practice began in the late 1970s, when a crystal form of the drug was created by mixing cocaine hydrochloride with ammonia or ether. (Ether was more frequently used than ammonia.) Now freebase cocaine can be produced simply by using baking soda and water, rather than the ether.

Ether is volatile, and early freebasers, in heating it, risked explosion. Richard Pryor almost died from burns incurred by preparing freebase cocaine this way. Freebasers, however, ignored the risks. Freebase cocaine goes into the bloodstream via the lungs which is the most direct route to the brain and the most effective means of absorption. For addicts, the pleasure this produced easily outweighed the danger of explosion. Those who smoke cocaine will feel the effects of the drug in approximately five to ten seconds.

Some medical professionals believe that smoking cocaine is more addictive than snorting because of its immediate effect. According to Charles R. Schuster, Director of the National Institute of Drug Abuse, animal studies have shown that as drugs are administered more slowly, animals find them less rewarding; presumably, the high becomes less intense (Holzman).

Originally, the freebasing process purified the cocaine. This is no longer true since different adulterants are now used. All of the "caine-based" adulterants (lidocaine, procaine, tetracaine, benzocaine and butacaine) are not burned off when the cocaine is smoked.

Cocaine vapors cause serious damage to the lungs and also harm the upper gastrointestinal tract. In addition, the speed and thoroughness with which freebase cocaine invades the system creates risks of its own. Cocaine overstimulates the heart while constricting the blood vessels; freebase cocaine magnifies both these conflicting effects, creating the chance of fatal heart or lung failures.

Freebasers usually buy the cocaine by the gram or fractions of a gram. They learn how to freebase from friends or books, and buy their equipment at stores specializing in drug paraphernalia.

Freebase houses sprang up when freebasing involved dangerous chemicals and required the use of extra paraphernalia; the houses supplied the necessary water-filled glass pipe and propane torches. Some addicts still frequent the houses simply because the work is done for them there and they can socialize with other addicts. The houses are located mainly in ghettos or other urban areas where freebasing is common.

4. Smoking/Crack

Crack is actually freebase cocaine with one important distinction — it is prepackaged, with no processing to be done by the user. Crack is sold already in the form of chunks or pellets, not powder. The crack smoker will feel the effects of the drug in the same amount of time that the freebase smoker will, in approximately five to ten seconds.

Crack is easier to use since the dealer has already prepared the mixture and sells it ready-to-smoke in tiny vials. The drug can be used in any kind of pipe and no other paraphernalia is needed.

Crack usually contains more adulterants than powdered cocaine. Since it's sold in chunks, the purchaser is looking at the drug's size, not tasting for quality. Bulk becomes important. It is initially less costly to purchase cocaine as crack, since it costs from $5 to $10 for one vial (approximately 1/10 of a gram) as compared to $75 or more for a gram of cocaine. But the long-run cost of a habit is probably about the same, as it seems that smoking cocaine is more addictive than snorting it.

Crack smokers experience the same physical side effects as freebasers (described in above section). Crack users will also frequent freebase houses that have now become crackhouses.

5. Smoking/Basuco

Basuco smoking is the least known, least expensive and least used method of using cocaine. Basuco, a paste derived from coca leaves, is usually mixed with marijuana or tobacco and then smoked. The paste, the cheapest form of cocaine, is often used in Latin America. Basuco represents the first step in processing cocaine; still holding lead and petroleum by-products, it is considered "dirty." On top of the health problems they share with freebasers, basuco smokers face additional hazards from their drug's contamination. People who have smoked basuco report that it tastes much like gasoline.

THE ADDICTION PROCESS

Cocaine addiction is different in several ways from other drug addictions. First, sedative or opiate (alcohol or heroin) abusers have usually developed a physical tolerance for the drug that causes physical withdrawal when they stop using it. Standard detoxification procedures include medication with sedatives. These drugs are decreased gradually to ease the pain of the withdrawal period.

Most treatment centers and hospitals do not use sedatives to detoxify the cocaine addict because they don't seem to ease the detoxification process. Recently, scientists have begun using drugs such as bromocriptine at Fair Oaks Hospital (Gold) and impripimine at Columbia-Presbyterian Hospital (Holzman) to curb the cocaine addict's craving. However, it is important to remember that it has not been demonstrated that these drugs do alleviate withdrawal symptoms.

Cocaine and particularly crack addiction can develop in months; by contrast, addiction to alcohol or heroin usually requires years of use. Cocaine addiction is also more immediately disruptive to the addict's life because of the bingeing pattern that swiftly empties out his or her physical, mental and financial resources. The financial aspect is critical: the habit becomes an expensive one very quickly.

Most cocaine addicts cannot be around the drug without using it until it's gone; the bingeing seems to begin by itself. As we have said earlier, users binge in hopes that more cocaine will give them back their initial euphoria. They also want the cocaine to lift them out of the depression (crash) that using the drug created in the first place!

Euphoria becomes the pot of gold at the end of the rainbow. Lisa, a recovering user whom we will meet later, describes a typical experience:

> Cocaine made me feel beautiful and powerful . . . This is what I had been looking for all my life . . . The cocaine gave me confidence, it made me feel accepted, it diminished and minimized my fears . . . On cocaine I was invulnerable; nothing could touch me.

Many cocaine addicts choose friends who use cocaine and avoid those who do not. They may miss appointments because cocaine use has taken precedence over other activities. The drug becomes the center of the addict's life. But, like other addicts, the cocaine user rarely recovers his or her early euphoria. As Lisa recalls:

> All those wonderful feelings happened in the beginning and became less and less frequent as I continued to use cocaine.

One characteristic of cocaine addiction is paranoia. For example, the football star Thomas "Hollywood" Henderson describes in his book, *Out of Control*, how he kept cocaine in his uniform during games because he believed that the FBI was pursuing him and would search his locker.

Some cocaine addicts will do anything to get the drug – lie, steal, cheat, even prostitute themselves. The drug's effects can also cause users to join in sexual activities that normally they would not have considered. Women may seek friends and/or lovers who can supply them with the cocaine, often choosing drug dealers as boyfriends. Lisa recounts what happened to her:

My main purpose in life became the attainment of cocaine. I would practically do anything for it. Toward the end [of cocaine use], I was involved with a cocaine dealer who abused me physically. I didn't care as long as he gave me my cocaine.

Some addicts will isolate themselves when cocaine no longer functions as a "social drug." The addict does not want to bother with people; most of all, he or she does not want to share cocaine with them. Freebasers, especially, tend to be isolated: after all, freebasers rarely smoke cocaine on the dance floor. If the addict becomes paranoid, the paranoia will heighten the social isolation. Paul, another recovering addict, describes his experience:

My only companion was a girl with whom I was living, and at this point of my addiction I had totally shut out all friends and family, never leaving the house for any reason whatsoever. I had food and drugs delivered because my paranoia was so great that I didn't dare to venture out. I was totally distrustful and afraid of anybody and anything.

Most addicts come to hate themselves. They have broken their own moral codes, have violated their values and have destroyed relationships with loved ones. They have enormous guilt and are greatly confused. At this stage, the addict is financially and emotionally bankrupt.

The real problem is that they still do not realize why. MOST ADDICTS DO NOT BELIEVE THAT COCAINE ADDICTION IS CAUSING THEIR PROBLEMS. THEY THINK IT IS SOMETHING ELSE, THAT THEIR PROBLEMS ARE CAUSED BY OUTSIDE SITUATIONS. We hear addicts cry with despair that their life is in turmoil because they have no money. They moan because their problems are caused by their spouse, employer, family member or friend. Jack describes what he thought:

My world was crumbling. My friends were in prison. I had very little money left. I was forced to sell my last external bit of self-esteem, my Jaguar, to raise money. I also got rid of furniture, paintings and televisions to raise money. It was a bit like playing Monopoly when you have to sell off your hotels at

10% of what you paid for them, just to stay in the game. I was severely depressed, but yet it never occurred to me that cocaine was a problem, that I was an addict.

This inability to see the root of their problems can cost cocaine addicts their spouses, jobs, families or friends. They may end up in jail, treatment centers or psychiatric hospitals.

Families, friends and employers can also fail to see what cocaine is doing to a user. Education about cocaine addiction is required to stop the cycle by awakening the addict and those near the addict to his or her problem and to the possibility of a cure. There are unmistakable signs of cocaine addiction that are physical, behavioral and psychological. When one becomes aware of the signs and symptoms of cocaine addiction, then the addiction cycle can be stopped. We have listed the signs and symptoms in the following pages.

Physical Effects of Cocaine

There are physical effects that result from cocaine use, most of them caused by the drug's stimulant effect. These include:

- dilated pupils
- tiredness from staying up all night
- headaches from sleeplessness, not eating or cocaine use itself
- decreased appetite, with weight loss
- dry mouth and nose
- bad breath, frequent licking of lips because of a dry mouth
- hand shaking
- convulsions from too much cocaine stimulation

When users snort cocaine, they will often suffer from:

- nose bleeds
- runny nose
- chronic nose/sinus problems

When users smoke cocaine (freebase or crack), the effects will include wheezing and coughing. If users inject cocaine, they will have needle-related symptoms, mainly abscesses.

No one can use cocaine regularly and remain unaffected; the

habit affects the user's behavior sooner or later. It is usually through behavior that one can spot a cocaine user. Not all of the following behaviors only happen with cocaine use, or even drug abuse. They do indicate a real problem, which needs to be addressed.

Behavioral Effects of Cocaine

- rapid mood shifts and swings
- blaming others for actions
- nonsensical excuses for poor performance
- memory loss
- loss of concentration
- anxiety
- irritability
- new compulsive behaviors (foot tapping)
- temper tantrums or rages

Cocaine use has psychological effects as well. These effects can sometimes be confused with the symptoms of other problems. As with behavioral symptoms, these signs are serious and need to be addressed, no matter what the cause.

Psychological Effects of Cocaine Use

- depression
- despair
- suspiciousness
- paranoia
- panic
- hallucinations
- delusions

REFERENCES

"A Clue to Cocaine Craving." Science Watch. *The New York Times*, 22 Sept. 1987:C3.

Fischer, A. "A Shock to the Heart." *Redbook*, Nov. 1986:88-90.

Gold, Mark. *The Facts About Drugs and Alcohol*. New York: Bantam Books, 1986.

800-Cocaine. New York: Bantam Books, 1984.

Gold, Mark, Verebey, Karl. "The Psychopharmacology of Cocaine." *Psychiatric Annals* 14(10) 1984:714 723.

Hall, James N. "Cocaine Smoking Ignites America." *Street Pharmacologist* 9(1) 1986.

Henderson, Thomas and Knobler, Peter. *Out of Control: The Confessions of an NFL Casualty.* New York: Putnam Publishing Group, 1987.

Holzman, David. "Crack Shatters the Cocaine Myth." *Insight* June 1986:48-51.

Kerr, Peter. "Anatomy of the Drug Issue: How After Years, It Erupted." *The New York Times* 17 Nov. 1986:A1,B6.

Lee, David. *The Cocaine Handbook: An Essential Reference.* Berkeley, California: And/Or Press, Inc., 1981.

Weitz, Alan. "Cocaine: A Pretty Poison." *Mademoiselle* Mar. 1985:176-177.

Chapter 3

Cocaine Addicts: Who Are They?

Cocaine addicts come from all walks of life. They are young, old, female, male, white, black, Hispanic, heterosexual and homosexual. They come from small towns and large cities. But while their stories may have different beginnings, the endings are always the same. Cocaine addiction robbed them of their lives, financially, emotionally, mentally and spiritually.

The following stories represent a cross-section of cocaine addicts, now recovered from their addiction. While their anonymity is preserved, they welcome the opportunity to share their stories in the hope that they may help someone else.

LISA

Lisa, a vivacious, slim blond, is eager to talk. She wants to share her experiences as a cocaine addict, and how these experiences affected her life. She emphasizes that she believes her cocaine addiction was part of her compulsive personality.

* * *

In retrospect, I realize I was compulsive before I ever started taking drugs. As a child I craved candy—anything sweet. When I was four years old, I ate a bottle of orange flavored pills the doctor had prescribed for my mother's morning sickness. I stole her favorite mints; I would eat as much candy as my little mouth could devour.

I was also addicted to books—fiction. I read and read and then I fantasized. I didn't like my own life; I wanted someone else's. I wanted to be a character in one of my books where everyone lives happily ever after. I was not a happy child as far as I can remember. I worried a lot. I realize now that much of this had to do with my parents. I don't blame my parents for my problems but I do see how their own lives affected mine. It didn't help that we moved frequently throughout my childhood and I was always the new kid on the block. I remember always thinking there was something wrong with me, that I was different from other people. It was as if I had some deep dark secret.

When I finally had my first drug, I was a prime candidate for full-blown drug addiction. We were living in Paris and I was fourteen and miserable which in itself is not so unusual. Taking drugs was the "cool" thing to do. I desperately wanted to be accepted so I smoked dope (marijuana) and took acid. This continued throughout my teenage years. It got to the point where getting high became my main focus. I didn't feel comfortable if I wasn't high. I constantly felt afraid and out of place and the drugs calmed those fears temporarily.

When I was eighteen, I moved to New York City and it was there that I was introduced to cocaine, the drug that almost killed me. I wanted to be a model and snorting cocaine made me feel beautiful and powerful. I was in the proverbial fast lane of city life and I thought, "This is it, this is what I've been looking for all my life." The cocaine gave me confidence, it made me feel accepted, it diminished and minimized my fears. On cocaine I was invulnerable; nothing could touch me. It was like that in the beginning. Cocaine quickly assumed importance in my life. I lost interest in modeling and became involved in abusive and destructive relationships with men. My main purpose in life became the attainment of cocaine. I would do practically anything for it. Toward the end I was involved with a cocaine dealer who abused me physically. I didn't care as long as he gave me my drugs. I had cocaine-induced convulsions and rarely ate or slept. It never occurred to me that I might have a problem. I felt there was something intrinsically wrong with me and the only way I knew how to handle it was to hide it.

I did have moments of clarity between binges where I would see what I was doing to myself. Occasionally I went to my mother's house in Connecticut and dried out for a few months at a time, but I always went back. I didn't know how to live without cocaine. My family was terribly worried and tried to talk to me but I laughed at them. Any time I talked to my mother, she told me I was going to die.

The last year of my drug taking was horrendous. I had to have cocaine upon waking or I couldn't get out of bed. I was paranoid and thought people were following and spying on me. I imagined that the telephones were tapped. I trusted no one. I was having violent fights with my boyfriend. I no longer enjoyed doing cocaine but I had to have it. It had become as important as breathing. I felt I couldn't live without it.

When I was twenty-eight years old, I lay on my bed in my small apartment and finally came to the conclusion that I had a problem. That problem was cocaine. I remember thinking that my life was always going to be a constant search for coke. I knew I had to do something or I was going to die. My friends had given up on me, my family barely spoke to me and even my boyfriend was tired of me. I called my mother and asked her if I could come home. She said I could if I would agree to talk to someone about my drug problem. I had been seeing psychiatrists for years, but they had just prescribed sedatives for my anxiety, which compounded my drug addiction. This time I went to a drug rehabilitation hospital and talked to a woman who helped me to recognize my addiction. I spent five weeks at this hospital where I was introduced to a Twelve-Step program and taught about drug addiction. Quitting cocaine wasn't physically painful, but, the psychological effects were devastating. All the feelings I had been stuffing with drugs for so many years began to surface and I couldn't deal with them. When I left the hospital, I continued to take cocaine for another eight months. The drug had lost its magic, though, and I now knew what I was doing to myself. I would snort lines and feel terrible. I envied the people I knew who were able to go through life without it.

Almost three years ago, I suddenly decided to get straight. I was sick and tired of being sick and tired. It was a crucial decision. It was the most difficult and courageous act I've ever done in my entire life. After almost fifteen years of fairly consistent drug-taking, I stopped. The real difficulty was dealing with who I was underneath years of taking drugs. I was frightened and confused. I didn't know how to get up in the morning without cocaine, much less live day to day. I didn't know how to socialize, how to have a relationship, how to function normally without cocaine.

Quitting cocaine meant starting over. It meant leaving behind people, places and things that had anything to do with my old life. It meant a lot of fear and pain. Above all, however, it meant the possibility of a healthy and joyous life free from the nightmare of cocaine addiction. With the help of a therapist, my family, a Twelve-Step program, physical exercise and my own inner strength, I have been free of cocaine for three years. Although it is sometimes hard, it is always interesting.

JACK

Jack has a ready laugh, and a quick wit that belies a seriousness about his life. As Jack's story will attest, Jack has not always been able to laugh. Quite the opposite, Jack had very little to laugh about, much less smile.

*   *   *

I was a late bloomer; I didn't start drinking on a daily basis until I was thirty-three. I snorted cocaine a year later, and injected it a couple of years after that. I was arrested after seven years of using drugs. I didn't tie it all together until a year and a half later. Cocaine was the cause of my criminal, financial and emotional difficulties.

I know now that my need to escape began real early. My original drug of choice was my ability to shut down emotionally and live in a fantasy world where I had been duly elected beloved emperor . . . where everyone was willing to love me unconditionally and do things "my way."

I was married in 1965, right after I passed the Connecticut Bar Exam and started practicing law. Every morning I was filled with feelings of anxiety which to me were overwhelming. My need to be perfect and to be loved created a great deal of inner tension and a friendly pharmacist turned me on to barbituates without a prescription. I used these on a daily basis for fifteen years, swallowing over one hundred milligrams a day at the end. Because they made me too mellow, the same pharmacist supplied me with amphetamines. Each day became a ritual of getting the right balance of "ups" and "downs" into my system so I could cope. I couldn't deal with the pressures of marriage so I spent four nights a week in my law office, working until midnight. Usually, my wife would be up and very angry at me for working such long hours. Unable to handle her anger, I began leaving my office at eleven p.m., stopping off for two or three vodkas at the local bar. I drove home feeling wonderful. My wife would still be awake and angry but now it didn't phase me. The lesson was indelibly stamped on my brain. I COULDN'T CHANGE REALITY, BUT WITH DRUGS I COULD CHANGE ME.

When I left the practice of law and my marriage, my first venture was to purchase a pharmacy. My world of pills expanded. Soon afterwards, I sold the business and built a medium-sized chain of discount eyeglass stores. I left the day-to-day management to others because of my inability to cope with stress and my fear of failure. I also stopped working because of my new-found love, cocaine, which was taking more and more of my time. It had become a full-time career.

The first time I did cocaine was at a disco one night when a friend offered me some. She told me it was a subtle drug and I didn't notice anything special, just that I seemed to sober up from the alcohol I had been drinking. I tried it again the next night. I hadn't been drinking. This time I started to feel in a way that I would try to recapture daily over the next seven and a half years. I experienced feelings of euphoria, self-confidence and power which I had always looked for. And since I wasn't drinking, there was no sloppy behavior, vomiting, or loss of control. I also noticed that lots of very attractive young women liked cocaine. And when I played the cocaine Pied Piper, they followed me home and into bed. Today I know that many men and women who become addicted to cocaine also become addicted to sex and I was no exception.

Within a short period, my whole life became centered around cocaine. It became my lifestyle. I owned a large waterfront home and encouraged various cocaine dealers to live with me. Getting caught up in the dealing end of the business, I now became the money man behind several cocaine transactions, all of which proved to be unprofitable. In the meantime, I wasn't showing up to my office until after four p.m. each afternoon, because of all-night cocaine parties. My money was rapidly running out, not only because of cocaine usage and drug deals, but to subsidize my business ventures, which were now losing money. I became a master of self-deception. It was just too painful for me to acknowledge that I was becoming a financial failure.

I was now doing cocaine around the clock, starting with the two lines next to my alarm clock which I laid out before passing out. My ability to converse was limited to "coke" talk; the price, flake or rock, various testing methods, and who was dealing the "primo." I started hanging out with cocaine smugglers who carried guns, so I purchased one and slept with it under my pillow. I took greater risks. When one of the gang I hung around with was arrested, I wrote an indignant letter to the Drug Enforcement Administration on my legal stationery, demanding to know whether they had anything on me. Not real smart!

Paranoia became my middle name. Discovering that I was under investigation, I sold my home and moved twenty minutes away. The profit on the sale of my home gave me an extra eighty thousand dollars to support my addiction. I was as reckless after I moved, openly snorting cocaine in restaurants, bars, men's rooms, while driving and in movie theaters. I attracted the normal crowd of cocaine ladies who were willing to give me the adoration and sex I needed in exchange for a few lines.

By mid-1980, I was spending about two thousand dollars a week on cocaine and couldn't subsidize my faltering business ventures. I had learned how to mainline cocaine from a friend whose father was a doctor. I reasoned that it was almost like a doctor taught me, so this was all right. I was always depressed and often felt suicidal. Sleep would come only after downing a quart of vodka and various sleeping pills, tranquilizers and hypnotics. Money was running out; I had gone to the limit with every bank that would have me. I was starting to get my own mother to invest in fictitious business ventures to support my drug habit.

My world was crumbling. My friends were in prison. I had very little money left. I sold my Jaguar to raise money. I also sold my furniture, paintings and televisions to get cash. I was severely depressed, yet it never occurred to me that cocaine was the problem, that I was an addict.

On February 14, 1981, I was reading about Thomas "Hollywood" Henderson in the local sports section of the newspaper. A former all-pro linebacker with the Dallas Cowboys, Henderson became the first NFL drug casualty to go public with his cocaine addiction. When interviewed, he stated simply: "Because of cocaine, I've lost family, friends and career." A flashbulb went off in my brain. For an instant I was restored to sanity. This was my moment of clarity. I got in touch with a psychiatrist and six days later he got me into a two-month treatment program. Today I am sure that if I didn't stop using cocaine and stay stopped, I would have been dead within a year.

I jumped into recovery with the same enthusiasm and drive that dominated my cocaine addiction. The seductive "white lady" had betrayed me. Intuitively, I knew I had a mission in life: to stay off the stuff, all stuff, and to help others who had also been betrayed by the "harmless" white powder. I followed the suggestions of my treatment center and went to at least one Twelve-Step meeting every day for two years. I didn't drink or do any other drugs for fear of going back to cocaine. In a couple of years I was able to accept that I was also an alcoholic.

I have learned to live a substance-free life "one day at a time," as they say. It has not always been easy. For the first year I didn't date because I just knew a woman wouldn't be interested in me. After all, I didn't have cocaine or the material trappings which had comprised all of my self-esteem. However, gradually, as my self-love grew, I started going out with women and enjoying them as people, not solely as bed partners. Financially, it is often a struggle, but a day at a time, I have a nice roof over my head and eat well. I managed to hold onto the one eyeglass store and it provides a good living for me. Although I can easily fall into the workaholic trap because I am such an obsessive person, money no longer holds the same value for me. My life, rather than being "thing"-oriented, is now people-oriented.

I am blessed today with wonderful friends. Like myself, they are all recovering people. I have worked hard to clear up the wreckage of my past. My oldest son graduated from college this year and we have a wonderful relationship. For the first time I am learning what a father is supposed to be and we work hard to understand one another. I know I've been blessed with a second chance and for the life of me, I don't understand why. I just accept this gift that God has given me with gratitude. I know that it all hinges on my willingness to stay clean and sober and help others to achieve the same freedom. I choose to try to live by spiritual principles today . . . honesty, unselfishness, purity and love. When I don't succeed, I don't beat myself. I just do the best I can . . . a day at a time.

AMI

Ami has a great amount of insight and is not afraid to express her feelings. Now in her thirties, Ami went through a lot to get where she is today. Even though it has been a hard struggle, she feels it has been worth every minute. She shares her story so she may help others in their struggle.

*　*　*

I always felt that I had a fairly normal upbringing. Born and raised in suburban Connecticut to an upper middle-class family, I was the youngest of four daughters and was born much later than my sisters. As a result, I always felt isolated and missed interrelating with siblings closer to my age. As a child I was shy and withdrawn. My parents were not particularly affectionate and I was left on my own a lot. I grew up with the knowledge that I was a mistake. I was jealous that my sisters experienced a sense of family life prior to my birth. I was envious of the families of my peers that appeared to be solid and cohesive. In my loneliness I spent a large amount of my time absorbed in fantasy play.

During my junior high years I made a conscious decision to change. Always feeling that I was missing something, I hated being me and I created a false self that was the opposite of my personality. The new me was bold and cynical. I created a self that could not be hurt. During these years I began experimenting with liquor and cigarettes. I never liked the taste but I enjoyed the fact that I was doing something dangerous and forbidden. I tried pot for the first time in the ninth grade and felt nothing, but this didn't stop me from trying it again and again.

The summer following ninth grade, we moved to St. Thomas and there I became the star I always wanted to be. People gravitated to me. I was no longer the little girl with braces and acne. I looked great and was up for anything. I particularly enjoyed the attention I got from men.

I tried acid that summer and loved it. It was the ultimate escape. Every night I would sneak out of my house and hit the bars, dance until dawn, and sneak back in. Alcohol gave me the bravado I needed and filled up that empty space inside. Without it, I was nothing. I continued using acid and alcohol through high school. On weekends I would spend all of my $5.00 allowance on a tab or two of acid.

When high school ended I set up housekeeping with an alcoholic boyfriend. I became a bartender and took great delight in drinking all my mistakes. I liked being a bartender because it made me the center of attention. It was during this time that I was first introduced to cocaine. I didn't feel it at first but after I tried it four or five more times I finally felt it. When I did, I knew that I had found what I had been searching for all this time. I felt omnipotent. Cocaine gave me the confidence I lacked. It made me witty and vibrant instead of self-conscious and insecure.

At the time, cocaine was very expensive and I swore I would never buy it. I soon found ways to use and abuse people to get cocaine.

Shortly after this I moved to New York and began attending art school. I had a friend who was a pot dealer at the time but soon increased his business to include the more profitable cocaine. He gave me lines on occasion that I would do and then get very creative and work on my art projects. At the time I could still turn it down if I knew I had to get to bed early to attend a morning class. However, my appetite for cocaine increased rapidly. I began dating the guy that dealt to my friend. I then started dating the guy that dealt to him, working my way up to the higher echelons of the drug ladder. I remember my first real "all nighter" where I exclaimed that I had never felt better in my life. I felt incredibly euphoric and loved everybody and the world. When it came time to crash, it was the day I was supposed to register for my third year of art school. I decided I had had enough of school and decided to move to Key West where there would be plenty of drugs to quench my voracious appetite.

In Key West I began hanging out with Cubans and others involved in the drug world. I romanticized that they were like modern day pirates. Cocaine had become the motivating factor in my life. Soon it got too "hot" in Key West and I returned to New York where I began doing intercontinental drug runs for drug dealers. They would pay me generously for my trips. Doing runs made me feel powerful and important. People on both ends would be happy to see me because I would be delivering either drugs or money. I was getting the attention I craved. What I didn't realize was that none of this was real. No one really cared about me. I had no real friends. This glamorous life was short-lived because the drugging was taking its toll and I was beginning to act hysterically. The dealers no longer wanted to do business with me.

I then moved to San Francisco where I soon discovered the needle. I began injecting cocaine, which caused me to become instantaneously addicted. I fell in love with the rush. During this time I had no real relationships of any depth. I became more and more isolated. I loved shooting coke because I was in control and I didn't need anybody. I would do — and did — anything for cocaine. I had a short stint in New York where I worked as a receptionist in an S & M parlor where I could act out all my sado-masochistic fantasies. I began hanging out in the punk underground scene where flirting with death was fashionable and I was accepted. I began to overdose on a regular basis. I couldn't hold a job. I worked as an exotic dancer to support my habit.

At the end of my drug-taking, I weighed ninety-two pounds. I was gaunt and came down with hepatitis several times. On my last run I had not fully recovered from a bout of hepatitis, but I continued to use. I suffered a partial stroke in my face and developed Guillain Barre syndrome, which attacks the central nervous system. I lost all feeling in my limbs and lay helpless in Bellevue Hospital for the next three months. I couldn't walk or talk. Cocaine had totally damaged my nervous system, and, to this day I am not fully recovered. I had gone about as low as a person can go.

It took all this plus one more run after I recovered to convince me that I might have a problem with drugs. My best friend talked me into attending Twelve-Step meetings. Although I fought it tooth and nail, I finally got it. It was very difficult for me because I could not imagine my world without drugs. I felt totally stripped of my defenses. In time I relearned how to live and began to feel that I might be worth it. I am forever grateful to my higher power who believed in me when I hated myself. I don't know why I was spared and others were not. I saw many good friends die from this disease. My main priority today is to remain drug free. I do this by being honest with myself and nurturing myself. I have to have faith and trust in God's will because the future is out of my hands. All I can do is live up to my highest potential and be there for people when they need me.

I have accomplished many things in sobriety. I went back to school and finished my B.F.A. in graphic design. I earned a Master's degree in Art Therapy and am presently engaged in a clinical psychology program that will enable me to be licensed as a psychotherapist. I worked as therapeutic director in a convalescent hospital and hope to start a practice focusing on compulsive disorders. I owe all of my success to the Twelve-Step programs and have learned not to fear but to respect my addiction.

TOM

Today, Tom is a warm, sensitive, caring man who exemplifies what a life without drugs can do for a person. He is a far cry from the man he used to be when he was getting high. Tom shares what life was like for him.

* * *

After twenty years of drugging and drinking, rehabs, jails and programs, I found myself at the age of thirty-three once again sitting in a rehab. At thirteen years old I started smoking reefer. By the time I was twenty-nine I had gone through barbituates, heroin, acid, methadone and was smoking cocaine. It was as if hell was breaking loose.

For so many years I'd lived in a prison within myself. I always felt that externals like money, a condo, a car or a good job would make me feel better about myself. I was wrong because I had them and I lost them as fast, feeling worse about myself. Now I can see that all of these objects are important, but not as crucial as what's inside. When I was in the last rehab, and the drugs and alcohol were taken away, I was like a frightened child. For so long I had played many, many roles and there I was sitting with myself, with no roles left. I felt lost, hopeless, in pain, and almost suicidal. Why not? I smile about this now, not because it's funny but, because so many changes have taken place, on the outside, and on the inside.

For me, it's great to be able to walk in public without feeling afraid of people or of the world. Today I talk with people, go to work, smile and laugh and feel comfortable. I have true friends and I can be with my family without feeling guilty or like an outcast. I try to be there to help people, not to use them. The ability to love and be truly loved are the true gifts of sobriety. When I started using coke it was all in fun and I did not believe it was addictive. I began snorting it, feeling that if I shot it I would be a drug addict. That was fun for a while, until the paranoia started to set in. I began drinking a little more to calm my nerves. Then I found myself snorting throughout the day and night. I lived in the world of drugging. It was either copping the coke, dealing or just hanging around the bars. After a while I burned out my nose from using so much and a friend mentioned that I should try to smoke it. That's just what I did. At first I had some control but not for long. All I wanted to do was sit and cook and smoke. I just could not stop. It was an obsession that I never experienced. My world became a small room with a pipe and a fish tank.

In my first year of sobriety I lived in fear. I had to learn how to live without drugging or drinking and it was difficult. I never would have thought that my life would be what it is today and I thank God for it every day. It's been six years now since my last drug or drink and my story does not end here; it's just the beginning.

CLARISSA

While I was growing up, I was a true follower. I needed to be loved and I needed the approval of my peers. I thought very little of myself and depended on others to make me feel good inside.

Clarissa, casually attired in a pink sweatsuit, looked at the floor after saying this. A few seconds passed before she looked up, smiled softly and continued:

*   *   *

Life for me was relatively normal. Then my father became an international executive and we were transferred to Hong Kong. It was quite a shock, going from a small town to a large, foreign city.

I was sexually molested by a man who worked for the family there. He began molesting me when I was ten years old and continued to do so for about one year. I was so frightened. Even though I was scared, I was afraid to tell anyone. I felt that somehow I was responsible for his behavior, that it was my fault that this man was abusing me. I kept this a secret until I was twenty-five years old. As I look back, I can see that I used the alcohol and cocaine to anesthetize my memories.

After three years in Hong Kong, my parents divorced and we moved to Europe. I began to drink. I learned that male attention helped me feel better about myself. Having a boyfriend made me feel like a "whole person." I preferred older men, usually twice my age. I don't know if this was because I was searching for the father that I no longer had. I became a flirt — it was the only way I knew how to communicate. I felt lost if I did not have a man's arm around me. Needless to say, the girls didn't like me.

I moved a lot, but no matter where I was, I found drugs. I used cocaine for the first time in New York City.

When I fell in love with cocaine, I really fell. The world looked beautiful. I knew all the answers, I had control, I was euphoric. I loved the lifestyle of staying up late and going out all the time. I went out with men who could support me and my cocaine habit. Not only did I want cocaine, but also money and champagne.

I never ended a relationship with a man unless I had another one.

In this way I did not have any time alone. While I used cocaine and other drugs and went from man to man, I also was an achiever. I went to college, worked and moved around the United States. However, the drugs hurt me. For example, when I was twenty-three I was hospitalized for serum hepatitis which was associated with my cocaine abuse. I was disoriented most of the time. I had hallucinations and heard voices. I was paranoid and thought that all telephones, including public ones, were tapped. I thought invisible bugs were on my body and consulted several doctors to determine the cause. I coughed up blood, the direct result of cocaine use. Doctors told me to stop using cocaine, but I could not. I was so paranoid that I couldn't leave the house. I finally felt so desperate that I overdosed on some pills and was hospitalized. It did not stop me from using alcohol and drugs.

I was careless about where I went and who I talked to. I was beaten and almost raped. I did not think that cocaine or drug use was related to these events; I just made a "mistake" one night.

By this time I had no place to go. I had no friends or money, and I called my mother. My mother was an alcoholic who had stopped drinking a few years earlier. She took me to a detoxification center in New York City. I was twenty-five years old.

Asking for help was the start of a new life. I became educated about addiction. I learned that cocaine use was the cause of my problems, not the cure for them. As time went on, I began to realize that alcohol was also a part of the problem. I began attending some Twelve-Step program meetings and seeing a therapist. I was amazed that my drug taking had masked all my feelings.

The hardest issues for me have been the "female" ones. Using cocaine masked the pain I felt from the effects of sexual abuse. It became necessary for me to participate in therapy for victims of sexual abuse, to heal the wounds. I was promiscuous because it was the only way I knew how to relate to men. My needs were met by my sexual activity and it was difficult to change this behavior overnight. I learned, however, that I can support myself both emotionally and financially. I don't need men like I once did. I earn my living and I am proud of it. I get validation of who I am from myself. I am assertive and say no when I don't want to be with someone or do something. My freedom today is indescribable.

In looking back, I can see that food was my first compulsion. I began taking diet pills to lose weight, not to get high. My initial use of cocaine was also to lose weight; when I stopped using cocaine I was terrified that I would gain weight. I almost started using diet pills, which could have begun another addiction process or caused a cocaine relapse. Today, I am conscious of my weight, but not obsessed about it.

I never felt intimate with other women when I used cocaine, whether high or not. I saw women as my competitors and I was afraid that they would take "my" men. Today I have a strong network of women friends, which means a great deal to me and my recovery.

When I used drugs, I was not aware that my body gave me messages. I was out of touch and my body was so numb that when I began my recovery, I could not believe the physical changes I felt. I discovered that I had Premenstrual Syndrome and while under its effects I experienced severe mood swings that caused strong cravings to use cocaine. I also discovered that my body was sensitive to birth control pills since I became emotional and felt out of control. When I got high, I was unable to separate the PMS symptoms, the Pill's effects and cocaine's effects. Today I can; I take measures to alleviate my physical discomfort without using cocaine or other drugs.

Today I can face these and other painful issues. I feel differently now, about life, about myself and about the world. I understand myself and enjoy life. If I had looked into my future I would not have dreamed that this rich life was possible. I am so grateful and my enthusiasm for life is beyond my wildest dreams. I couldn't have asked for more.

TONY

Tony has never felt very good about himself. While his family had material wealth, there was not much emotional wealth. Tony did not feel "wealthy" until he used cocaine. Like many others, Tony thought cocaine would provide all the good feelings that he didn't have. It did, until the reality of cocaine addiction set in.

*   *   *

I am a middle child in a black middle class family. My dad was always at work when I was growing up and my mother pretty much brought me up. I never had much emotional support in my childhood; my father always told me I was stupid and my mother didn't know how to express love. We lived in a nice home and had a big white Cadillac. It wasn't as if I was materially deprived.

When I started in school I became a bad kid. I'd fight the other kids and distract the class. Academically, I did well enough to get by. Physically, I looked like a mess; I never combed my hair and I always had a runny nose. My mother made us go to church and I never understood what God was all about, although I did enjoy singing in the church choir. I loved baseball and gave it my all. I grew up like most other kids. My friends were very special to me. It may be that I was addicted to them.

My first drug was after my sixth grade graduation. My main man Stuart and I decided that we wanted to smoke some reefer. His sister smoked it all the time and we ended up buying a five dollar bag from her after getting ripped off by the brothers on the corner. We smoked the pot and drank a few beers and I felt like the Six Million Dollar Man. I felt great and wanted to feel this way all the time. Within two years I was getting high in the morning before school and staying that way all day long. My father always gave me money and I prided myself on the sharp clothes I wore to school. I considered myself a big shot. I wasn't able to talk to the girls sober but when I was high I could sell them the moon. The only problem was that pot and beer made my eyes red and my breath stink. It took away from my cool demeanor. I reached the point where I wanted to stop getting high. I was flunking out of school and I caught V.D. three times in one summer. I didn't feel like the Six Million Dollar Man anymore. I got straight for about a year. My family gave me a car, I got back into church, and my grades went up. I met my girlfriend, with whom I was madly in love.

Then one day I was introduced to cocaine and that was it, the wonder drug. I was told it wasn't addicting and I got it free from a friend in return for driving him around in my car. With coke I knew all the answers in school. My girlfriend didn't know I was using.

Shortly after graduation, I started working in an automobile manu-
facturing plant and it was great. I had the perfect job, a big income,
no responsibilities and drugs galore. Then my girlfriend and I broke
up and my heart was broken. I started sniffing, smoking and drinking all the time. I started hanging out with the "cocaine girls" and
soon I met the racketeers in the city. One man took a liking to me
and told me to come hang out more often. Soon we were best
friends and I had cocaine and guns to spare. I didn't like what I was
becoming so I joined the Army. I got into a lot of trouble and was
thrown out. While I was there I joined a drug program but I wasn't
able to stop using drugs.

When I got out there was a new drug on the street called crack
and I thought it was meant for me. I couldn't get enough. I was
driven to keep smoking it. I'd buy vials of it and promise myself I
wouldn't buy any more, but it was never enough. Even when I
bought jumbos it still wasn't enough. I was always trying to get that
feeling I got when I first smoked it, but that feeling never came
back. Even after it stopped feeling good, I couldn't stop and I
would have done anything to get it. I was spending all my money
hanging out with the petty drug dealers on the street. I was afraid of
being arrested so I decided to stop getting high. I entered my first
drug rehab.

They tried to tell me I had a disease and couldn't do drugs anymore. I didn't stay there long. I was determined to beat this on my
own. In three weeks I was back to coke sniffing and smoking like
never before. My family was furious and I went back to another
rehab. This time I made friends and was exposed to several Twelve-
Step groups and realized I was like these people. However when I
got out, I started getting high again. Finally I quit, locking myself
up with my then-pregnant girlfriend. I dried out and became afraid
of myself and my disease. I left the house only to go to work. One
day I went to a Twelve-Step meeting. I was told to go to ninety
meetings in ninety days, get a sponsor and to listen to suggestions.
It's been four years now since I got high and I think I've stumbled
upon an unshakeable foundation for life. There has been growth in
every area of my life. I've been blessed with a healthy daughter.
I've had no trouble with the law and I believe in a power greater

than myself. I'm at peace with the world today and at peace with myself. I don't need drugs to be happy.

FRAN

Fran speaks about her addiction to cocaine and where it took her. In her early thirties, Fran is enthusiastic about life, and her joy for living is a far cry from when she was addicted to cocaine.

*   *   *

If you looked at my life from the outside, everything looked pretty good. I was successful in my career, attractive and ambitious. In my early twenties, I was well on my way to being a respected speaker and performer in the hair industry. However, inside things were very different. I felt insecure, always needing approval from others, never feeling good about myself. I felt like a phoney and feared that someone would "find out" that I was not the person I appeared to be.

For many years I used drugs only to ease the anxiety I felt because I didn't know how to cope with my anxious feelings. I smoked pot in the evenings and if I couldn't sleep I took sedatives. I rarely drank and at first I used cocaine only for special occasions. I'm not sure exactly what happened or when it happened, but all of a sudden I found myself wanting more. Cocaine made me feel powerful, in control, confident. I could work harder and longer; I was more outgoing and, best of all, I stayed thin. I thought I had found the magical answer to all my problems. What was once used for special occasions became an everyday need.

This started a never-ending roller coaster ride of self-destruction. As my usage increased, I began to need other drugs to sleep. At the end it was a daily diet of cocaine, pot, sedatives and booze. I was always trying to find the right combination and amount of drugs to get the perfect high, which I never found.

My whole life began to fall apart; I went from one bad relationship to another. I began to isolate; I could not stand to be with people yet I was desperately afraid of being alone. I had panic attacks and was actually paralyzed with fear sometimes. The magical drug that once made me in control now controlled me.

It was not until I reached a point of desperation that I sought the help I needed. At the time I believed that cocaine was my problem and if I could somehow find a way to stop using, all my problems would go away. Through a Twelve-Step program I did in fact get sober. I also found that I had many other issues to work on besides the drug addiction. The real courage in recovery for me was to become willing to look at the issues that caused me to be so uncomfortable with myself in the first place. Until I could start to take a look at these problems I could never develop the self-esteem I needed to become the person I wanted to be. Using drugs caused problems in my life, but I came to realize I had some problems which caused me to use drugs. I had to take a look at my attitudes toward life and my belief systems. I always felt like a victim. Having been adopted, I had abandonment issues, feelings of never belonging. All of these issues manifested themselves as low self-esteem, fear of rejection and many other problems.

Through recovery in a Twelve-Step program I have been able to work on these issues. Recovery for me has been a lifetime spiritual journey of self-discovery. I'm slowly learning self-acceptance, self-love and self-understanding. Today my life is wonderful. I have very special people in my life who I care about and who care about me. I can take risks. Fear no longer paralyzes me. I am truly happy without cocaine or any other drugs.

RALPH

Ralph is as committed to his new life as he used to be to cocaine and other drugs. Ralph has beat the odds. A Puerto Rican growing up in Harlem, he has achieved a life he never hoped for. And Ralph is always glad to share his story.

* * *

In 1983 at the age of thirty-nine I committed myself to a detoxification center. I was in horrible shape, with no teeth and only the clothes on my back. For years I had been taking drugs and I finally admitted that I was a cocaine addict.

I am a Puerto Rican who grew up in a poor family in Harlem. By the time I was eleven years old everyone I knew was into drugs, alcohol and running numbers. I never felt that my family was close; my father was always working and my brothers called me names and slapped me. To prove myself I became involved with a gang and started using drugs. When I was fourteen I ran away from home and was arrested. After I was released from jail I never returned to my family and grew up doing what I wanted to. I believed I was unlovable and I pushed people away who cared about me. I felt lonely and what helped was drugs and alcohol. I still had dreams, however, and I finished high school in Puerto Rico.

When I joined the Navy, my drinking and drugging got me into trouble and I became violent. I managed to get an honorable discharge and returned to Puerto Rico to go to college. In college my drug use escalated and I began to do heroin and to deal. In the six years I was at college I lost both money and friends.

When cocaine came into my life, I fell apart. I began shooting it, spending a lot of money, becoming incredibly paranoid and always feeling lonely and scared. I tried to quit a few times but I always went back and always saying: "This will be the last time." I tried switching from cocaine to heroin when I realized what it was doing to me. I dealt drugs to supply myself and was arrested again, although I beat the case after a ten-month ordeal.

After I finished college, I decided to go to New York and start working. I hoped to return to my family but they decided to move to Puerto Rico and my dream of being with them again was delayed. I got a job as a token Puerto Rican with a college degree but because the salary couldn't support my drug habit, I quit and began dealing again. I ended up on a methadone maintenance program for nine years, sleeping in abandoned buildings, subways and parks. I ate in soup kitchens and felt lonely, scared and tired all of the time.

The night before I went to detox was spent shooting cocaine and sedatives. The next day my journey into recovery began. I spent a year in treatment and attended self-help groups. I found myself and discovered a God of my understanding. Today I can tell you that I stay clean one day at a time with the help of my self-help groups. I have a job, a home and a beautiful wife. I visit my mother every year and I have plans to see my brothers and sister after years of being estranged from them. I have developed a faith in religion which has helped me and continues to help me. I believe that this has all been made possible by the grace of God.

SYLVIA

Sylvia never felt like she belonged. She wanted to be American but her father insisted that she be the "perfect little Spanish girl." She tried, and at first she succeeded. She received good grades and she was active in school clubs. However, she also took drugs, and her cocaine addiction took her places no one ever thought she would go.

*   *   *

I had my first drink when I was eight years old and I immediately fell in love with the feeling of warm security that booze gave me. For the next seventeen years I chased after that warm feeling with many different drugs. Cocaine was the drug that brought me to my bottom.

Having been born in Cuba, I moved with my family to the United States when I was a year old. When I was four we settled in a small town in New York where we were the only Hispanics. My father believed that we were going to return to Cuba and insisted that we keep our Cuban culture alive. He was very strict and discouraged us from emulating our American friends. From the beginning I felt different, as if I didn't fit in, and these feelings of insecurity and inadequacy became worse as I got older.

Being the only Hispanics in a small town was difficult. It made fitting in very hard. My father became stricter and called my friends stupid and inappropriate, and I learned how to isolate to avoid these tirades. I tried to fit into both American and Cuban society, yet I felt like a misfit. Relief came in the form of the barbituates I was prescribed for menstrual cramps when I was thirteen. The barbituates were even better than that first drink. I went through high school stoned on barbituates, sedatives and pot. The drugs gave me that warm feeling that allowed me to stuff my painful emotions.

I started to deal to support my habit and the people I hung around with were drug friends. Life at home was a series of violent fights between my father and me and I started using more downs.

By this time I associated with people who lived in the drug world. This life appealed to me; the only priority was to get as high as possible. Despite my drug use, I still looked like your "average good kid." I was on the twirling squad, in chorus and I had good grades. Inside I was a mess and I believed that what was important was to get high. As long as I could keep up my facade, it was possible.

When I graduated from high school, I was very confused and decided college would solve my problems. I attended a small community college nearby since my father refused to let me go away. This, however, was not the solution and I started doing heroin and hallucinogens with a man I met.

My relationship with my father became worse and I ran away, living in the woods and at different people's houses.

Then I found men. I discovered that if I stayed in bars, I met men who gave me drugs and took me home with them. This eventually led to prostitution. I never thought that the sweet girl I had been would become a prostitute. My feelings of despair and self-hatred became harder to dull with drugs. I thought that the answer lay in moving away and starting a new life but that didn't work and after my parents were divorced, I moved back in with my mother. Speed replaced the downs I had been taking and then cocaine replaced the speed. During this time I suffered from severe guilt around having prostituted myself and the drugs helped numb the pain.

Once I started using cocaine my life became insane. On cocaine I could work, attend school and party full time. I associated with any man who was willing to provide me with cocaine. My desire for the drug was insatiable; I could never have enough. Once again I was prostituting and because I needed more and more, I often had more than one "boyfriend" at a time. I lied to my family and friends about what I was doing. I was insulted if they ever questioned me about my drug use. Everything looked fine from the outside; I was working and going to school — how could I possibly be using? This was my denial; addicts didn't have cars or jobs.

As my drug use increased, so did my insanity. Along with my cocaine use I drank and used pills. When my friends thought I was becoming "too wild," I changed friends. Eventually, I started associating with people who were worse than I was. This somehow made me feel better.

My bottom began when I found a drug dealer who gave me cocaine in return for my company. In this relationship there was no fooling myself or anyone else. I was in it for the cocaine. My friends no longer wanted anything to do with me and I spent my days working and my nights partying. This man taught me how to freebase and I became obsessed with it. I would take hits off the pipe at my job, in the bathroom or driving in the car. I didn't care who saw me; I needed the freebase. After a while I could no longer drive to work because of the paranoia. I thought there was someone in the back of my car. I quit my job because it interfered with my getting high. I entered into another relationship with an old friend who gave me as much cocaine as I could base. I spent all my time freebasing with him. I knew what I was doing but I couldn't help myself. I felt totally alone and desolate and there was no turning back. Who would ever want me after?

Help came in the form of a television announcement for a cocaine hotline one day when I was desperately trying to find some drugs. I looked at it and continued trying to make contact for my freebase. It was as if God was trying to get through to me because the ad came over the T.V. again. I thought they might give me drugs and tried to dial them but, ironically, I couldn't spell cocaine. I alternately dialed my dealer's number and the hotline number and eventually got it right. A man answered and asked me for my name and where I lived. His questions scared me and all I told him was that I might have a small problem with cocaine. He gave me the addresses of some Twelve-Step program meetings and the first meeting he told me about was in my town. I went into a deep paranoia imagining that the phone had a T.V. camera. After I hung up I ran around insanely pulling down the shades and trying to see if anyone was watching the house.

After trying to reach my connection, I began dressing for the meeting, still intending to get high if I could reach my connection. It took me all day to get dressed; I wanted to look as normal as possible; I was still trying to pretend I was all right. I ended up in front of the meeting place and as I was trying to decide whether to go in, a man asked me if I was looking for the meeting. I was shocked and upset that I might look as if I had a drug problem yet I went in with him. Inside were a group of men sitting around a table and I immediately thought I was going to be raped. However, I was treated like a queen; they used kid gloves and urged me to come back. A couple of days later I returned and I kept coming back and eventually understood that this was what I had been searching for all my life. Here, people loved me for who I was in spite of what I had done. I found hope and I learned that I had the disease of addiction but that recovery was possible. I learned to trust and to love.

Today I have a job that I love and enjoy, friends who love me and a husband who understands my past and doesn't hold it against me. Best of all, I have me, something I never had before.

SEAN

Sean is charismatic and outgoing, the "life of a party." Despite great suffering throughout his life, he has an enthusiasm and joy that can't be missed. He smiles winningly and is willing to share his life story with others so they may be helped by his experiences.

*   *   *

Not only do I have a problem with cocaine and alcohol, but I am also gay, bulemic, a clinical manic-depressive, as well as an adult child of an alcoholic, and an incest survivor.

I was born in Cranston, Rhode Island in 1948. Both sides of my family are riddled with substance abuse. I was sexually abused by my grandfather as a young child until my father finally caught him and threw him out of the house. This issue was never dealt with until I was thirty-six years old. I spent my adult sexual life looking for older wealthy gentlemen who would abuse me, never understanding the pattern I followed, until I was in recovery.

As a child I was prescribed various medications for my strange behavior. I always felt I had to prove myself to my parents and apologize for something I didn't understand. I developed a severe stutter and would hide in the basement playing Broadway records over and over.

As the years went on, my family became increasingly dysfunctional, but I was lucky to have a wonderful English teacher who got me interested in acting and theater. She arranged an audition for me with a local theatre company and I was hired as an apprentice, which changed my life. By the time I was seventeen, I had hooked up with a well known burlesque show and had become a musical comedy stripper. I worked under false I.D.s and made a lot of money.

The few times I tried drinking, I had blackouts. At twenty-one, I was prescribed sedatives and immediately fell in love with them. It answered all the pain I held inside. The hole was filled. I was then introduced to Black Beauties because I was so tired from the sedatives. When people asked me what my drug of choice was I always answered "YES, anything, anytime, anywhere." I even took drugs that I didn't like, as long as I didn't have to be me.

At this point in my life, both my parents died from substance abuse. My dad died of cirrhosis of the liver and my mother died of wet brain. I swore this would never happen to me, but it almost did.

I got a job teaching in a high school with emotionally disturbed teenagers. This was to be a career that I would work in on and off for many years. During this time I was diagnosed as a manic-depressive. I was prescribed anti-depressants and was warned to stay away from all recreational drugs and alcohol. Naturally, I didn't believe what the doctors told me, and I created my own living hell. When I was down, I craved ups and vice versa. It became a nightmare, to say the least.

I was first introduced to cocaine at my job as a burlesque performer. Someone spelled my name with it on a makeup mirror. I loved it. It made me feel so up and carefree that I forgot all my medical problems. I felt I could run for president and win. Later that night I wound up in the psychiatric ward. I was then given more prescribed drugs. My medical drug intake increased as my cocaine abuse grew out of control.

My twenty-year career as a burlesque performer quickly came to an end. I lost urinary and bowel control. I wasn't able to sing or dance, let alone memorize lines.

The Actors Equity Association helped place me in a rehab in New York City. I had to agree to stop all medication until they could figure out my true personality and the extent of my manic depression. At this point I would have sold my soul to get clean.

I was more sick in recovery than in my drug-using days. My medical bills were so expensive that I lost all of my money and wound up on welfare and food stamps. I continued treatment in an eighteen-month aftercare program. My counselor introduced me to a woman, who was sober for several years. She became my best friend and taught me how to do simple jobs that I had always done on drugs. She accepted me for just me. The doctors put me back on medication. It wasn't easy but I began to get a glimpse of what sobriety was. I wanted it badly and hung in through the bad times.

I retired from stage work and went back to school to renew my teaching license. I left a nine-year relationship. I waited until I was two-and-a-half years sober to move to San Francisco. I became self-sufficient. Today at five years sober, I have my own studio apartment that I alone pay for and I am in graduate school working on my Master's degree in Rehab education. Most importantly, I work in an adolescent rehabilitation center, teaching school and running a theatre company called *Clean and Dry Playhouse*. Was it all worth it? Yes, every painful emotion brought me into the world of reality and sobriety. My advice to the addict is — Hang in, don't give up, it does work. Without the Twelve-Step programs, I would not be able to share my experiences with you today. All I can say is do what I have done; GO FOR IT! STAY CLEAN!

Chapter 4

Addict Questionnaire

DO YOU HAVE A PROBLEM WITH COCAINE?

1. Do you use cocaine until there is none left?
2. Would you use more cocaine if you had more money?
3. Do you think you'd be less productive without cocaine?
4. Does cocaine make it easier to socialize or work?
5. Have you tried to stop using cocaine?
6. Do you need more cocaine than before to get high?
7. Do most of your friends get high?
8. Have you missed an appointment because of cocaine use?
9. Have you stayed up all night doing cocaine?
10. Do you use cocaine in public places like restaurants, restrooms, cars or planes?
11. Do you think about getting high frequently?
12. Do you use cocaine when you are alone?
13. Do you try to get more cocaine when your supply ends?
14. Did you take people's cocaine without their permission?
15. Have you bought cocaine with money that should have been used for something else?
16. Has anyone said that you may use cocaine too much?
17. Do you say you use less cocaine than you really do?
18. Do you avoid your family or friends?
19. Are you ashamed by some of your actions?
20. Are you having financial difficulties that could be related to your cocaine use?

If you have answered yes to 3 or more of the questions listed above you may have a problem with cocaine.

Chapter 5

The Adolescent Cocaine Addict

Experimenting with drugs, including alcohol, is a rite of passage for many American teenagers. For some, this is just a phase; for others it is the beginning of a journey into addiction. Amy's experience is typical.

*   *   *

When I was twelve, I began experimenting with drugs. I discovered that when I was high, I could avoid the unpleasant feelings of insecurity and shyness, which all kids have. I did not realize the necessity of having these feelings to become an adult. Even if I did, I probably wouldn't have cared since my main concerns were to be popular, "cool," and to belong. Using drugs gave me a crowd to hang out with and made me feel like I was witty and popular. I believed that drugs were the answer to all of my problems. Actually, they caused more problems than I ever imagined.

Between the ages of twelve and fifteen, I tried a variety of drugs. I began smoking pot on a daily basis at thirteen and continued to do so until I was twenty-one. I was first introduced to cocaine when I was fifteen. This was in 1978 or so, when cocaine was getting a lot of attention from the media. It was portrayed as a nonaddictive and very glamorous drug. At least this was how I thought it was being portrayed. Some older friends showed me how to snort coke. It is very difficult to explain the feeling you get from the first time you use cocaine. For me, it made me feel confident, popular, attractive, witty and convinced me that I belonged to the "in crowd." Cocaine gave me everything I thought I ever wanted. At the age of fifteen it was difficult to get the money I needed for the cocaine, so I stole from my parents. For example, I would take my mother's jewelry and sell it. My parents confronted me with my stealing. I would deny it, even when I was caught.

At this point, my "partying" and my friends were more important than anything else. I went to school in order to see my friends. I rarely attended classes and was dropped from the honor ones. When I did show up for class, I was high and obnoxious. I was suspended from school approximately once every three weeks. My parents did not know what to do with me. They were strict some of the time and lenient at other times. My cocaine use was erratic. I would go on coke binges for several months, and then would switch to other drugs for a few months. I did everything I could to find the people who had access to coke, and I made sure that I was around them when they were using it.

After high school I went to a small community college in New York. By now my parents were divorced and neither of them trusted me with keys to their homes. They could not trust me since I was caught stealing from them. I had also spent my student loan money on cocaine. Although I felt I did not know how to make new friends at college, I always managed to find the drug users. To make sure I always had cocaine, I started spending time with older men who had both money and cocaine.

I heard about freebasing and decided that this was much "cooler" than snorting coke. I then met some people who lived in New York City who introduced me to freebasing. I thought I had arrived! This was where I was meant to be! I had heard that when you freebase you get an incredible rush from the first hit. Afterwards you keep smoking the base (cocaine) to recreate that feeling. Once I was introduced to that pipe, I could not think of anything else. It was all that mattered to me.

When my friends weren't available, I went to vacant buildings in the Bronx to buy coke. I was now in a new world — one with guns and people who used code names. I knew I was in over my head, but whenever I got nervous about going to the Bronx, I would take a hit of coke and my fears would disappear.

After freebasing for a while, I tried to end my life by swallowing a large quantity of pills. You see, one of the characteristics of cocaine use is that after the initial feeling of euphoria, you become very depressed. To lessen the depression, I drank or used sedatives.

I thought my life was useless, that I was a hopeless human being, destined to be miserable.

The suicide attempt made me take a long look at my life, and I decided that the cocaine had something to do with my depressions. My answer was to switch addictions, so I stopped using cocaine. For the next six months, however, I increased my use of marijuana, sedatives and alcohol.

This didn't work and after another suicide attempt, I called a psychiatric hospital near my college. *I still did not think I had a drug problem*; I was convinced that I had a mental illness. After all, you have to be insane to be twenty-one, a junior in college and obsessed with ending your life. Luckily, the hospital I called had a drug and alcohol program.

In the hospital I was confronted with my drug use. I was forced to examine my attitudes and behaviors and their relationship to drugs. The staff emphasized that addiction was not a moral issue; I was not a "bad" person. I was informed that addiction is a disease. I had a choice about what I was going to do about it. I found out that addiction not only affected me physically, but mentally and emotionally as well.

Part of treatment in the hospital included attending various Twelve-Step meetings. Most of the people at these meetings were much older than me. They had been drinking for twenty to thirty years and had not used drugs. I could not make the connection that I was like them. Then I heard a woman speak who had used cocaine and had many similar experiences to mine. I spoke with her and suddenly felt that maybe there was hope for me. I was not destined to be miserable; I could be happy someday!

It has been over four years and I cannot describe the difference between the person I was then compared to who I am now. I have done a lot of emotional growing that I never did when I was a teenager. I am expressing my feelings for the first time in my life. I am learning about love; how to give it and receive it. I managed to squeeze a lot of misery into a short time. Now I have a lot of living to do.

I know that I cannot use any type of drug. I need the support of other recovering addicts to stay clean. They understand me because

they have shared my experiences, if not physically, then emotionally.

I would really like to emphasize that cocaine is an addictive drug.
It will take everything from you. This drug takes prisoners and I
was one of them. I am no longer that prisoner; I am free today and it
feels great.

ADOLESCENTS AND COCAINE:
WHY COCAINE?

Why are today's adolescents using cocaine? When we talked to
adolescents and professionals, they provided some interesting ex-
planations. Most agreed that teen use of cocaine is primarily because cocaine, particularly crack, is now cheap. Teenagers can obtain crack at or near school for $5 to $10 a vial. Crack's availability
and cost are not the only reason for its use. After all, a bottle of
wine costs about $2. First, cocaine is an easy drug to hide, easier
than alcohol or marijuana. It is easily hidden in a pants pocket or
purse. The teenage cocaine user can usually drive a car, attend
classes and eat dinner with the family without being suspected of
using cocaine. Second, cocaine doesn't smell like alcohol, and it
doesn't cause hangovers. Unlike alcohol, cocaine is neat; you don't
slur words, and you don't fall down.

Finally, cocaine gives adolescents the feelings they desire:
power, confidence, sex appeal, and intelligence. Adolescents crave
these feelings because they often feel powerless, insecure, dumb
and not very sexy.

Adolescent girls told us that they like cocaine because it helped
them stay thin. Thomas White, Director of the Jamaica Community
Adolescent Program (JCAP) in New York City dismisses this ratio-
nale as an excuse to use cocaine.

Crack also appeals to adolescents because it is a quick high that is
painless and neat. Adolescents do not like to use needles or create a
mess. This dislike of mess and needles once prevented teens from a
quick addiction to cocaine that occurs with intravenous use of cocaine. Crack, which offers a fast and intense high, has changed the
pattern of teen cocaine use.

Cocaine is the "in" drug of the 1980s. According to Ellen More-house, Founder and Director of Student Assistance Services of Ardlsey, New York, cocaine reflects the values of today's society.

In the 1970s, marijuana was the "in" drug. During those years, people were "laid back." They wanted to be mellow and relaxed. It was important to be a "free spirit." The popular music was folk singing. Joni Mitchell and Joan Baez were the singing stars. There was a tendency against materialism. People wore low-cost jeans, especially white painter pants. Marijuana, as a drug, represented these values. The marijuana effect, initially, was one of relaxation. It was inexpensive because it would grow anywhere.

Society no longer holds these values. It is a different story in the 1980s. Status counts, and to count, one needs to be on the fast track, be a "mover and a shaker"; be on top of things. Materialism is "in," as evidenced by the almost universal sight of designer jeans and name-brand running shoes. One must look good, be "hot." The pop star Madonna represents these values — she is hot, sexy, and materialistic. Cocaine fits these values. It is a stimulant, providing the confidence and energy to be a mover and shaker on the fast track. It is more expensive than marijuana, representing class and quality.

SPECIAL EFFECTS OF COCAINE USE ON ADOLESCENTS

Children and teenagers do not understand the long-term effects of cocaine use. Teenagers think about the present; they do not realize people burn out on cocaine and that cocaine is different from other drugs. Cocaine creates addicts far more quickly than alcohol, marijuana or heroin.

Teenagers aren't entirely responsible for this misperception, according to Nancy Kessler, private therapist and Supervisor of Training and Clinical Practice, Student Assistance Services, New York:

The most frightening aspect of adolescent cocaine use is the adult perception of cocaine. Many adults do not perceive cocaine as very dangerous. This is a grave mistake since cocaine is very destructive. I meet parents who think that cocaine can be "snorted once in a while" without any damaging effects. There is no safe way to use cocaine since the potential for addiction is greater than with any other drug.

Cocaine's physical and psychological impact on anyone is severe. Its impact on adolescents is even more dangerous because an adolescent is still developing.

Not only are teens still developing physically and emotionally, but some important decisions need to be made. For example, teenagers are expected to make career decisions: choosing a college or trade school to attend. Adolescents who use cocaine are unable to plan ahead; cocaine is their primary concern. Since they are not concerned about tomorrow, they will binge more.

A tendency to binge and the lack of income help destroy the teenage cocaine user's life. The need to finance their cocaine habit can drive them to betray their values and instincts, especially when they steal from their family.

We know many parents who refused to believe that their teens have lied to them or stolen money from their wallets. They are shocked and refuse to admit that their child has become a "criminal." This denial is understandable, but it does not help the adolescent. Helping the adolescent requires confrontation about their drug use and treatment for it.

Teenagers cannot progress through a normal adolescence when they are preoccupied with cocaine. Adolescence can't be relived, and so teenage cocaine addicts require assistance in developing skills that they never learned. Additionally, because they have usually sacrificed their values, they suffer a loss of dignity and self-respect. These also need to be bolstered in treatment.

Many professionals believe that cocaine use most often follows from use of alcohol and marijuana. Madelyn Venner, Executive Director, National Council on Alcoholism and Chemical Dependency, says that she has not encountered an adolescent who "just used cocaine.'' We agree because, usually, an adolescent will experiment with alcohol and marijuana first and then move on to cocaine.

Cocaine's impact on teenagers can be easily detected by anyone who watches them. We have developed a list of symptoms that indicate cocaine use.

If you suspect cocaine use, remember that it is something to worry about. It is a serious problem and will not go away after a lecture.

SIGNS OF ADOLESCENT COCAINE USE

Are you confused? How do you determine when a child is going through normal adolescence versus abusing cocaine? When we asked the experts, they unanimously agreed: it's easy to tell the difference once you know what to look for.

In addition to the physical, behavioral and psychological effects of cocaine use that are described in the ''Cocaine and Cocaine Addiction'' chapter, there are several behaviors that are unique to adolescent cocaine use. They include the following:

At Home with Family

- change in attitude toward parents, siblings, rules
- withdrawal from family functions
- stays in room alone, often for long periods of time
- blames others for irresponsible actions
- lies
- irregular eating habits
- irregular sleeping habits
- verbally abusive
- physically abusive or violent
- defiant (breaks curfew)
- becomes more secretive

At School

- sudden drop or gradual decline of grades
- cutting class(es)
- ending sports or other extracurricular activities
- acting disrespectful towards teachers
- defiance towards rules
- increase in disciplinary actions
- sleeps in class
- inattentive in class
- preoccupied with drug culture (music, posters, T-shirts)

With Friends

- changes attitudes toward non-drug using friends
- changes peer groups with little interest in old friends
- makes new friends who are strangers to parents
- associates with older people
- fights with peers

WHAT THE FAMILY/PROFESSIONAL CAN DO

There are solutions to an adolescent's drug addiction. The following are do's and don'ts for families and professionals when dealing with a possibly addicted adolescent:

Do:

- Wait until your child is *not* under the influence of drugs before confronting him or her
- Keep in mind that you did not create your child's problems — he or she did
- Provide and consistently maintain, consequences for drug-induced behavior, such as restitution for property loss or destruction
- Keep communication lines open by keeping the focus on "I" and not "You"
- Realize that your child's drug abuse is not a matter of weak will power

- Remember that the way the child acts when using drugs is not an indication of a lack of love — the drug addiction causes dramatic and usually negative personality changes
- Respect your child's privacy by not eavesdropping or searching their room when they are out; monitor behavior and use examples of his or her behavior as indicators of drug abuse
- Listen to your child and talk honestly with him or her
- Seek information and support regarding drug addiction

Do Not:

- Make excuses for abnormal or unacceptable behavior
- Bail the teen out of messes (school, legal or interpersonal problems)
- Allow the adolescent to keep drugs or drug paraphernalia at home
- Permit drinking at home or at the wheel. For teens, alcohol is as illegal a drug as marijuana or cocaine. Furthermore, allowing drinking sets up a double standard and sends a contradictory message
- Allow the addicted adolescent to attack and abuse you; or attack and abuse the adolescent
- Act as if all is well when it is not
- Refuse professional help for various reasons ("what would the neighbors think," "we can handle it ourselves")

These guidelines can help stop the addiction cycle. The adolescent must face the destructiveness of the addiction. Only then do addicts begin to acknowledge their problem and accept treatment.

Addicted adolescents often act self-sufficient and unapproachable. They work hard to keep adults at a distance and to avoid questions about their cocaine use. Addicted adolescents may tell parents and professionals what they want to hear. This may suit the adults, since they may not want to acknowledge the problem.

It is the rare adolescent who seeks help on his or her own accord. Treatment centers and outpatient clinics are full of adolescents who were forced into treatment. Fortunately, once the adolescent is educated and helped, many go on to a drug-free life.

Professionally guided intervention by the parent is one way to help an adolescent. Interventions have a high success rate in getting the adolescent into treatment. (Intervention is discussed in more detail in the Family chapter.) Finally, the family (and professional, if appropriate) must become familiar with the disease of chemical dependency. They must learn the signs and progression of addiction as well as the means to recover from it.

Treatment Options

Families cannot help their teens face their addiction and recover from it alone. They must consult a professional, preferably, a team of professionals. We recommend that a family consult their local alcoholism/drug abuse agency for a referral. It is beneficial to seek assistance from a team of specialists that are trained in chemical dependency and who are linked to the mental health community. If the problem is not chemical dependency, they then can make the appropriate referral.

Adolescents often need in-patient treatment if they do not have the support of their families. They also may need in-patient treatment if they live with family members who abuse alcohol and/or other drugs. It is also necessary to remove adolescents from their drug-using peers. There are some, but not many, out-patient programs for adolescents that provide all-day treatment.

Twelve-Step Programs for Adolescents

Twelve-Step programs provide an excellent means for adolescents to stay away from cocaine and other drugs. Participation in a Twelve-Step program such as Cocaine Anonymous, Narcotics Anonymous or Alcoholics Anonymous can make all the difference to recovery from addiction. The crucial component of these programs is a social network of drug-free teens. This is crucial for a teen's development as a source of peer approval and acceptance.

Adolescent Recovery

The chances for recovery for an adolescent are excellent if the adolescent receives good treatment, participates in a Twelve-Step Program and has the support of family. You must note that adolescents often relapse (use drugs again) more than adults. They have less to lose and are more vulnerable to peer pressure. They have less control over their lives. They cannot change neighborhoods or schools as an adult can. There are also developmental issues for the adolescent, such as rebellion against authority. They are still developing interests and need to replace drug use with activities that many teens consider square. The importance of drug-free friends cannot be emphasized enough.

Most adolescents strongly resist participation in Twelve-Step programs. This is mainly because these programs are geared for adults and most adolescents would rather hang out with their friends. A good therapist/counselor will guide the adolescent to a group where there are a lot of young people. A good therapist will also translate the adult language so the adolescent is not turned off.

SCHOOLS

Schools can play a crucial role in the adolescent use, abuse and recovery from cocaine addiction. If a school denies a drug problem among its students, then the students will continue to use drugs. A program of intervention is necessary to stop the addiction cycle in the schools.

Many school officials believe that it is not their responsibility to raise children. Their role is to educate children and blame parents for any behavior problems. This attitude fails the students. Because of the length of the school day, teachers and school officials often see more of their students than the parents.

Many teachers believe that kind words and a hug are the answer for a teen's addiction. True, these are part of the answer, but nothing more. We must treat teenagers who are suspected of cocaine use the same way we would treat adults who are suspected of cocaine use. They must be confronted with the facts and consequences of their behavior. It is not helpful to excuse their behavior; it is not helpful to the parents, school or the teens.

Schools can exert pressure for drug abstinence. This can be accomplished by bringing chemical dependency experts into the schools to design programs. Also, teens love to listen to stories:

having recovering teenage addicts speak can produce a positive impact. By allowing Cocaine Anonymous, Narcotics Anonymous or Alcoholics Anonymous to hold after-school meetings will assist those who are trying to abstain from drugs and alcohol. Teenagers need places near at hand, places where they don't need to be driven to build a drug-free social network.

Chapter 6

Adolescent Questionnaire

FOR THE TEEN:
DO YOU HAVE A PROBLEM WITH COCAINE?

1. Would you use more cocaine if you had more money?
2. Have you tried to stop using cocaine?
3. Do most of your friends get high (on anything)?
4. Have you stayed up all night doing cocaine?
5. Have you bought cocaine with money that should have been used for something else?
6. Do you say that you use less cocaine than you really do?
7. Have your grades gone down in the last 2-3 years?
8. Have you cut classes more than 3 times in the last year?
9. Have you dropped any extracurricular activity? (sports)
10. Have you been suspended or expelled from school?
11. Have you been in trouble with the law?
12. Do you break your curfew or stay out all night?
13. Do you have new friends who party more than your old ones?
14. Have you sold any of your or your family's possessions to get money?
15. Have you taken money or jewelry from anyone in your family?
16. Are you less interested in religious activities, like church?
17. Have you lost weight?
18. Have you sold cocaine or other drugs?
19. Do you look forward to when you will do cocaine?
20. Do you wish that you could stop using cocaine?

If you answered yes to more than 3 of these questions, you may have a problem with cocaine or another drug.

Chapter 7

Relapse and Relapse Prevention

Webster's New Collegiate Dictionary (1983) describes a relapse as "a recurrence of symptoms of a disease after a period of improvement." It goes on further to describe it as "the act or instance of back-sliding, worsening, or subsiding."

There are no definite causes for a relapse. Many people have lost jobs, have had loved ones die or have weathered other set-backs without using cocaine again. People who start using cocaine again may not even be consciously aware that they are making excuses for this use. In fact, most cocaine addicts who relapsed agree there were clear signs before their relapse, but that they just didn't see them. We see this when looking at Paul's story.

* * *

My first experience with cocaine occurred during the early years of my marriage. Like most addicts I've encountered, I started using it socially with my friends. I fell in love with the feeling of euphoria and omnipotence it gave me. The progression was rapid, leading to a seven-gram-a-day habit from a quarter-gram within one year. I should have recognized that my cocaine usage was different from others because my wife never used more than four lines each time and never more than once a week. My denial was so strong that I thought that she was the one that was abnormal, not I. My marriage, my work, and my relationships with other people worsened at an increasing rate.

At the time of my divorce, I was totally alone and I was introduced to freebasing. The insidiousness of freebasing was twofold over snorting; the initial high was much more rapid and greater in intensity and the resulting depression was equally dramatic. One change that was noticeable to me was that I was able to stop for a few days between snorting, but when freebasing it was one continuous nightmare without food or sleep for days. My only companion was a live-in girlfriend. At this point of my addiction I had shut out all friends and family. I never left my house for any reason. I had food and drugs delivered because of my paranoia. I didn't dare venture out. I distrusted and feared anybody and anything.

At the time, my mother was dying and rather than deal with those feelings, I opted to freebase. It was shortly after her death that I made a promise to my family to enter a rehabilitation center. I remember being petrified of the unknown, and not believing I could live without cocaine. I had a positive experience at my first rehab. At the end of thirty days I felt like a new person, cured from my addiction to cocaine. I ignored any suggestions to enter a Twelve-Step program because I felt so strong.

I picked up cocaine within one week of leaving rehab and the progression took off just right where I had left it. Three months later, I entered my second rehab, this time for sixty days. Again, feeling cured, I ignored any suggestions to get involved with a Twelve-Step program or aftercare. Within two weeks I was back exactly where I left off. I decided that I needed a geographical cure, so I moved to a new house a little farther from home. This did nothing but further alienate me from my friends and family.

My paranoia led to boarding up all the windows of the house. I would not stay in any room of the house without my pipe, my torch and my gun. At this point, a family intervention, the threat of commitment and the threat of having a court-appointed conservator for my trust fund forced me to go into rehab once again. I left that rehab after four days, once again, swearing that I was through with cocaine. Naturally, within a short time I was right back to where I had left off; my addiction was rampant.

I decided that another geographical change would cure me so I hired a driver and rented a Winnebago. I took my girlfriend and one ounce of coke and headed for California. I finally ran out of coke in Wyoming. Within four days, I called my dealer in Connecticut and had him fly an ounce to Cody, Wyoming. When I reached Las

Vegas, word came that my father was dying and I should return home at once. I chartered a jet, returning home looking like a homeless bum. Obviously, in my present state, I was of little help, and no consolation to my family or my father. The fear of his ensuing death only pushed me further into my cocaine use. About one week later he died and I did not attend his funeral because I was unable to put my pipe down.

The guilt and shame that I felt were even greater than that which I felt after each relapse. I was devoid of any self-esteem. Yet it was several months, following a serious car accident, before I decided to try rehab once again. I went to a prestigious rehabilitation center in Southern California which had a reputation of helping chronic relapsers. I fell in love with the people and the patients from the start. It was there that I began to listen to the ideas of the Twelve-Step programs. I attended many meetings in the various Anonymous programs. For the first time I began to deal with my feelings and emotions.

This time I followed the suggestions given to me and went to a halfway house and continued my meetings. When I finally returned to Connecticut, I was clean and sober for over a hundred days for the first time in twenty years. I decided that I felt strong enough to continue my recovery on my own.

Within three weeks without meetings and aftercare, I was back to a five thousand dollar a week habit. The pain, guilt and remorse was stronger than it had been before. I had also emotionally, physically and psychologically deteriorated. Fortunately, this time I was brought to my knees within a very short time. Unfortunately, my bottom encompassed being arrested for possession of cocaine and my car was seized following another car accident. The greatest humiliation was having my name in the newspaper, where it was read by family, friends and acquaintances. Little did I realize at the time that this was a blessing in disguise.

I then entered my last rehab, this time beaten and with a willingness resulting from despair greater than ever before. I believe that my changed attitude and extreme emotional bottom allowed me to stop fighting the suggestions given by other recovering addicts and alcoholics. When I left that rehab, meetings were no longer an option: they were a necessity for continuous sobriety. It was not long before I was comfortable within the walls and among the people in the recovery fellowships.

I never thought that after twenty years of addiction I would ever celebrate one year of continuous sobriety. To my amazement, this came true. Unfortunately, having met this goal, the attitude that accompanies addiction compelled me to pull away from the program. I had come to believe that my two higher powers—first, God, and secondly, the friends that I had come to love very deeply within the fellowship—would and did restore me to sanity in my sobriety. It should not have, therefore, surprised me that upon pulling away from both the Twelve-Step program and from God, that a relapse was coming.

I had always denied my alcoholism and after sixteen months without alcohol or drugs of any kind, I decided to drink. When people speak of hitting a bottom, one thinks that a bottom is about the amount used, or the length of time that one is using. This time my bottom occurred after three drinks. I finally realized that a drug is a drug, even if it is in liquid form. The guilt and shame that I felt, the feeling of being alone, and the loss of self-esteem were even greater than I'd ever experienced before. I felt alienated from the people who I had come to know and love in the Twelve-Step programs. I was so afraid of rejection, judgement, and the loss of their love that it took six weeks for me to share my relapse at a meeting. Although painful at first, I was at once reassured of the unconditional love and forgiveness that I had always known with these people.

I have often heard addicts say that if they had enough money, their addiction would not be a problem. I am living proof that all money facilitates is an even more rapid addiction progression. Even though there is no financial incentive to stop, the most important incentives, those of pain, remorse, insanity and self-degradation, are enough. I am deeply grateful to the Twelve-Step programs with which I am associated and most especially to those people within them whom I love and need. They have helped me to regain a loving relationship with my God, achieve self-respect and a well-being greater than I have known before in my life.

DRINKING

We have seen, time and time again, people who return to cocaine use because they started to drink, or continued to drink after they had given up cocaine. Many of these people did not believe they were problem drinkers, and perhaps some of them were not. However, the alcohol lowered their inhibitions so they didn't care about their abstinence from cocaine. Let's take a look at John's story as an example.

I stopped using cocaine when a crisis led me to the realization that it was killing me. I never felt that I had a problem with drinking alcohol and didn't consider drinking when I stopped using cocaine. I had not used any cocaine in four months when I was visiting an old friend. I was thirsty and asked my friend for something cold to drink. He said, "help yourself." When I opened the refrigerator, there were only some six-ounce mini-beers. I thought "I haven't had any alcohol in four months. What could possibly happen if I had just one small six-ounce beer?" Then I remembered someone telling me that a drink could lead me back to using cocaine. I thought about it and decided if I never liked alcohol, then I didn't have a problem with it. I'm drinking a beer because I'm thirsty, not because I want to get high.

With that, I proceeded to drink the beer and thought nothing more of it. An hour later, my friend and I went out for dinner. My friend ordered a drink, and I thought, "That beer didn't affect me so what harm would it do if I ordered a drink with dinner?" So I ordered a drink. After dinner I said to myself "I can drink, I feel good and I don't want cocaine. I ordered an after dinner cordial. I looked at my friend and said, "I've got some money. Why don't we buy a little cocaine. We'll just snort it, so we don't become compulsive like we would if we smoked it." After snorting for a little over an hour, I said, "lets get some more. We'll prepare it so we can smoke it." So we went and bought a large quantity of cocaine. When we arrived at the head shop to buy the paraphernalia, it was closed. By now I had such a compulsion to get high that I lost hold of my senses and grabbed a big rock to throw into the shop. All of a sudden I became clear, and in that moment of clarity I saw where that six-ounce beer had taken me. I put down the rock and I burst into tears. . . .

That was four years ago. I have not had a drink or a drug since that day. I learned that a drink, even for a person who doesn't have a problem with alcohol, is dangerous. It will affect clarity and judgement.

Others didn't go back to using cocaine but continued drinking, switching their addiction from cocaine to alcohol. They were not using cocaine any more, these people told themselves, therefore they didn't have a problem. The point is illustrated by Danielle, a petite, attractive young woman who had been using cocaine for five years. In her own words she'll describe what happened.

I got into serious trouble with cocaine use. I had to get treatment or go to jail. This worked because I was able to stop using cocaine, alcohol and all other drugs. I was able to show the court that I could be a law-abiding and productive member of society.

I found a freedom with ending drug use and looked forward to getting up every morning. I felt alive and happy. Slowly, however, problems began to occur; everyday problems that I wasn't used to dealing with straight. I was having financial difficulties, as well as job problems. I had never learned how to deal with stress, since I had always used drugs during stressful times.

During this time, a lifelong friend invited me to her wedding. I was thrilled about seeing all of my old friends. I accepted the invitation and looked forward to the big day.

The day before the wedding was tough. My boss said my performance was inadequate. I went home to find that the kitten had torn up my most beautiful plant. There were also bills that I couldn't pay.

However, the next day I was determined to have a good time. I was so happy to see all of my friends. Before I knew it, it was the moment of the toast. I had not even thought to ask for ginger ale instead of champagne. I said to myself, "What's one glass of champagne?'' I drank it and found that it helped to relax me, and my troubles disappeared. I thought, ''This is the answer. I don't need cocaine, I'll just have a drink once in a while to relax.'' I felt happy. I would drink in moderation and never touch cocaine again.

This worked very well for a while, although I had to be careful because my therapy group believed in total abstinence from everything. However, I knew I could control my alcohol use and keep it hidden from others.

As time passed, however, I wanted to drink more often, and had a hard time not drinking before group therapy. I began having just a couple of drinks before going to group, and would chew lots of gum to hide the smell. The group noticed a change in me, but didn't know why I was behaving differently. One night the group therapist smelled alcohol on my breath, and confronted me. I denied any alcohol use, got very angry and stormed out of the group. For the next two weeks I didn't go back to group and my drinking increased. My boyfriend caught me in a friend's kitchen, chugging some wine. I lied to him and cautioned myself to be more careful.

However, my use worsened in those two weeks and I almost lost my job. I realized that my life was unmanageable and all of the good feelings I had when I first stopped getting high were gone. I hated myself, I felt guilty and I couldn't stop drinking, even though I wanted to. I knew I had to make a change. I called my group therapist and asked if I could come back to group. I knew I could get the support I needed from them. I went back and asked for their help. I am now able to stay away from alcohol and all other drugs with the help of my group. I'm grateful to have learned, even if it was the hard way, that the only way for me to feel good and enjoy life was to stop using all drugs.

FEELING CURED

Many people believe that they are cured after receiving short-term therapy, either inpatient or outpatient. They feel that they will not use cocaine again and they have a strong resolve not to do so. One of the reasons they feel this way is that their therapy enabled them to feel in control of their drug use. Without the continuous positive reinforcement of therapy, however, it is easy to start using cocaine again.

We will see this illustrated when we look once again at some of Paul's story:

> At the end of thirty days in my first rehab I felt cured. I ignored any suggestions to enter an outpatient program because I felt so strong.
>
> I picked up cocaine within one week of leaving rehab and the progression took off just right where I had left it. Three months later, I entered my second rehab, this time for sixty days. Again, feeling cured, I ignored any suggestions to get involved with outpatient therapy. Within two weeks I was back exactly where I left off.

Paul repeated this experience.

> Coming out of another rehab, I followed the suggestions given to me. I went to a halfway house and continued my meetings. When I returned to Connecticut, I was clean and sober for over a hundred days for the first time in twenty years. I then decided that I was strong enough to continue on my own.
>
> Within three weeks without therapy and meetings, I was back to a five thousand dollar-a-week habit.

Paul's experience shows that recovery from cocaine addiction is an ongoing process. Furthermore, when a person tries to do it on his or her own, it will most likely result in a relapse.

PEOPLE, PLACES AND THINGS

People

A person who is beginning recovery from cocaine addiction will hear the statement: "stay away from people, places and things." This is heard in treatment programs, individual therapy and Twelve-Step meetings. It means those people, places and things that a cocaine addict associates with using cocaine. Jane's story demonstrates why:

> I knew that I had to stop drinking alcohol and using drugs, especially cocaine. I was going to therapy and attending Twelve-Step program meetings. I couldn't stop seeing my friends; after all they *were* my friends. So I would go to a meeting or to a therapy session and afterward, I would call up my friends. They would cop some cocaine and I would get high. I met people at the meetings who said "stop hanging around with cocaine addicts or you will continue to do drugs." They were right. Sometimes I would try to see my friends and not use cocaine, but that never worked. Every time I talked to one of my drug-using friends, I would get an urge to get high and all my best intentions went out the window.
>
> Not only would I hang around with people who used cocaine, I also went to bars and the streets where people got high. I always got high when I went to these places. I would get a certain feeling in my stomach and that would signal "get high" to me. I could not stop using cocaine as long as I saw my friends and went to the places where I got high. So I got high and spent my money and the money that I borrowed so I could get as much cocaine as I could. I felt terrible when the high wore off. I hated myself; why couldn't I stop? I did not stop getting high until I stopped seeing my friends.
>
> It was also necessary to avoid the street and bars where the drugs were. This was difficult at first but became easier as time passed. I was shocked that my friends did not call or try to see me. I realized that they were not true friends since they only wanted to get high with me. At first I was hurt, then angry, then relieved. I was relieved because I was not tempted to use cocaine again, by them at least. By staying away from them and the places, I got stronger and stronger so when I did run into them, I was able to say no to cocaine.

It is very difficult, if not impossible, to not use cocaine if one socializes with people who use cocaine or other drugs. It is hard to say no to cocaine when it is in front of you. That is one of the main reasons people start using cocaine again. Even if one does not use cocaine, why put oneself in the position of temptation? Often, recovering addicts feel that they have to prove that they can turn down cocaine or other drugs. It shows that they are strong, that they can do it. Instead, many give in to temptation. So what are recovering cocaine addicts supposed to do? They cannot live in isolation, or spend their remaining years without socializing. They must build a network of friends who don't use cocaine or other drugs. It is difficult to stay drug-free without supportive friends.

Billy explains how he did it:

> At first I resisted meeting new people. I thought they were dull and boring. However, I soon realized that I was scared to death of being rejected. What would I do if these people didn't like me? It was easier to stay with my friends who used cocaine and wouldn't reject me. The problem was that the cocaine was killing me, so I couldn't stay with my old friends. I knew that if I didn't make new friends I would use cocaine again.
>
> It had been a long time since I talked to people without the crutch of cocaine, alcohol or other drugs. It sure wasn't easy; but I did it because my life was at stake! I met people at meetings and I went to the movies and to dinner with them. Actually, I felt the safest with these people because I knew we were in the same boat. In time I was able to socialize with people who were not recovering addicts by practicing and forcing myself to go out with acquaintances. It worked, and I made new friends so I was not tempted to hang out with my old drug-using friends. By not hanging around with drug-users, it was easier not to use drugs!

Many cocaine addicts have urges to use cocaine when they see old friends. Many of them, like Jane, are unable to stop using cocaine until they separate from certain people. For some, this may even mean separation from the family, since it is common that families share addictions.

Most relapses occur because an addict has not stopped associating with people who use drugs. Some relapses occur because an addict encounters a drug-using friend and cannot resist the offer of cocaine. One must avoid the places where one can find drug users so the temptation does not happen.

Places

Places that can prompt cravings to use cocaine vary from individual to individual: for some it is a bar, or a neighborhood, or street; for others it is a baseball game or rock concert, for still others it may be clubs or certain restaurants. Clancy avoided many places because he was very susceptible to cocaine cravings.

> During the first few months, I had to stay away from a lot of places that would tempt me to use cocaine. At first I felt foolish; after all, I was an adult, I couldn't hide from life forever! I soon realized that I was acting like an adult when I avoided places that were dangerous for me. I stopped going to Yankee games because I used to smoke marijuana and drink lots of beers at those games. After getting high on marijuana and beer, I always bought cocaine, so Yankee games were a no-no, at least for the first few months.
>
> As someone who loved to dance, I really didn't want to give up the clubs. I had to, however, because I spent money at clubs on cocaine! And believe it or not, I couldn't visit my brother and his family for a while. My brother lived in a building where I used to buy cocaine and when I went to that building I was overcome by cravings to use cocaine. I explained this to my brother and we arranged to see each other outside of his home. It may sound silly, and I certainly felt silly, but by avoiding these places, I did not use cocaine.
>
> I also realized that by avoiding these places I was beginning to control my life. I was not at the mercy of these places where I felt tempted to use cocaine. By having some control I also realized that I had choices. I chose to avoid these places and I was not tempted to use cocaine. It became easier and easier, and after a while I automatically did not go certain places and it did not bother me.

Things

Recovering addicts must avoid or replace things that are associated with cocaine or other drug use. For instance, recovering addicts are strongly advised to throw away drug paraphernalia. There is no reason to keep drug paraphernalia unless one plans to use drugs. Here is what happened to Peter:

> I had been selling cocaine for quite some time and I had expensive equipment for testing and weighing cocaine. Someone suggested that I get rid of it because it was a reminder of my cocaine addiction. I thought, I'll hold onto it until I find a buyer. So I kept it with the intention of selling it. In the meantime, the equipment brought back strong memories of the past and I began to have cravings to use cocaine.
>
> Then I started to have financial problems. When I saw the scale I thought of all the money I used to make. Within a matter of time I was dealing cocaine to make money. I started doing a little cocaine. Before I knew it, I was doing more than I had ever done. My life became a horror. I am thankful that I was able to stop. I sure learned my lesson; I don't keep anything around that reminds me of cocaine.

Recovering addicts differ in the things they must avoid that tempt them to use cocaine. Rose Ann had to throw away her Sweet and Low packets because the white powder reminded her of cocaine. Dennis stopped taking inhalants for colds because it reminded him of snorting cocaine. For others it could be small mirrors, razor blades or sandwich bags. Troy talks about all the things he threw or gave away because of their associations with cocaine use:

> I couldn't believe it when it was suggested that I give my rock music collection to a friend. I was relieved, however, because I would get urges to use cocaine whenever I listened to that music. I thought, "My life is over, oh no, I am becoming old before my time." There was a certain sweatshirt that I wore when I smoked crack; it even smelled like crack! Well, that sweatshirt had to go and I threw that away. It was amazing how many things were associated with cocaine use and I reluc-

tantly gave them away. I am glad I did because I know people who have urges to use cocaine and because they have kept things that are reminders of their cocaine use. I believe that it is better to start a new life without drugs, and what better way to start it than by throwing away all the stuff that is associated with the old life.

Chapter 8

The Family

Janine de Peyer, MSW, CSW

In many ways, addiction is a family disease and needs to be treated on a family basis. In this chapter we will explore how.

We hear a lot about cocaine, and the painful struggle an addict faces in overcoming his or her addiction. People always want to know who addicts are, why they became addicted, and what they did about it. But what happens to the people who *love* these addicts?

How many people stop to think about the close family members and friends tied up in this struggle? What about the parents, spouses, siblings, friends, children, employers and employees of the cocaine addict? What happens to them emotionally, physically and mentally, as they watch their loved ones wrestle with addiction?

These are the important people behind the scenes. They are the ones who care, support, love and try to protect the addict from his or her own destruction. They are often the ones who suffer when the entire family savings go toward the use of cocaine. Sometimes they are business owners who are bankrupted by embezzlement of funds.

Perhaps the most painful situation is that of the parent, watching his or her child fall into addiction. Christine, the mother of a nineteen-year-old cocaine addict, describes her feelings when she discovered her son's problem:

Janine de Peyer, MSW, CSW, Clinical Social Worker, New York State Certified. Formerly Psychotherapist, Jewish Board of Family and Children's Services, New York. Currently Outpatient Family Social Worker, Smithers Alcoholism Treatment and Training Center, New York; Private Practice.

CHRISTINE

*   *   *

We call them "Dog Days" in New York. Hot, humid, sultry, with the smell of rotting garbage in the air. This was not the reason for the surge of nausea that overcame me. No, the cause was something far deeper, for my 18-year-old son, Pete, had confessed he was addicted to crack.

Actually, I had confronted him with my knowledge of his theft of my bank card. He had stolen nearly $3,000 from my checking account. Better yet, it was from my credit line, which left me with the responsibility of repaying what had become an unauthorized loan. I looked at him with disgust and contempt. Any pity I felt for him was obscured, at that moment, by the wish that he would die. Maybe then I could be released from the weight of the misery he had caused me.

As I sat in my apartment later, I began to rethink his and my life together. Our hardships had forged us into a closely knit, almost symbiotic family. As would any parent under this circumstance, I begged to know where I had gone wrong. Accepting responsibility for everything that occurred in our family was what my life was about.

Pete and I got off to a bumpy start — at the age of 17, while still in high school, I discovered I was pregnant by a friend of my boyfriend's (my boyfriend was away on active duty with the Army). This man was seven years older than me, and I chose not to tell him. Rather, I sought everything within my power to arrange an abortion (not easily done in the tiny town in Idaho where I grew up). Failing on that score, I tried to arrange to have the child and give it up for adoption — also to no avail. I then made the only other choice I could see for myself at that time. I married my boyfriend and hoped I could pass the child off as his. Naturally, with this less-than-idyllic beginning, that marriage ended eighteen months later. I found myself left with Pete, many bills, no education and no family support system. My family had long since turned its back on me, but I had been left with an overpowering desire to make something out of my life — and I would succeed.

Pete was an adorable baby, full of charisma and charm, and I worshiped him. Our early years together were good ones. Although I had to work two jobs to "make ends meet," I spent most of my free time with him. I was determined he would not suffer from the rough start we had. My ambition led me to move to California, where opportunities were better. I began attending college at night, while working a demanding job during the day. This necessitated leaving Pete with a baby-sitter for most of the day, and he began to develop a vivid imagination, spending hours in fantasyland. I thought his interest in fairy tales was endearing, until I discovered he had developed a habit of stealing.

He stole from stores, and later he stole from me, and the pattern was formed. I would deny he had done it, then beg him to tell me why. I would blame myself for my obviously poor mothering, and resolve to be a better mother until the next time. I accepted another high-powered job in Chicago, where the stealing continued. I traveled a great deal for business. On several occasions, unable to find a baby-sitter, I left him by himself overnight. He was only ten. His loneliness and fear of abandonment resulted in an even greater interest in fantasy—books, characters, movies and lies. We then moved to New York, where I set up a business of my own. I spent even more time away from him, working to try to achieve financial success and recognition. I hoped I could fill up the empty chasm caused by my own childhood experience of rejection and abandonment.

Pete was always a bright and gifted student, yet I regularly received notices of his behavior problems in the classroom. Either he would disrupt the classroom, or refuse to do his homework or, eventually, skip school. The parent/teacher conferences pointed out one fact that I could not accept: I made excuses for his poor behavior, and he took advantage of my fear of being an inadequate parent.

At times I did not perform my parental duties well—I used drugs, often in front of him. This certainly set a poor example of responsibility. However, I rationalized my own drug use by telling myself my own life was tough. Like my son, I also retreated into fantasyland. As I look back, the good times Pete and I had together always revolved around vacations and long weekends away. This was another example of our need to escape from a life that was difficult.

My business was high-pressured, and the anxiety of living in New York added to it. Also, I had numerous disappointing relationships with men, followed by periods of deep depression. Pete was always there to comfort me and wipe away my tears. He'd tell me, "It will be okay, Mommy." As he grew taller, I jokingly used to tell him I looked forward to when he was a little taller. Then he'd be able to escort me to all my social functions. I always had invitations, but I never felt I had a date. What a burden Pete had to bear!

Pete chose to go away to prep school, so finally I thought I'd have a life of my own. I realized one day that my loneliness was now being filled by ever increasing hours in my office. I lived for vacations when Pete would come home, for he was truly the man in my life. I can see now why he found drugs appealing. They were also readily available in his prestigious New England prep school.

Before long, the same problems he had faced in New York were surfacing there — I began receiving a litany of letters again describing his behavior problems. They complained of lack of discipline and refusal to do his homework. Eventually they decided not to invite him back the next year. All of my high hopes and aspirations for him were smashed. Somehow, I had felt that if he had the advantages of an Ivy League education, he would have an easier life. He would have entree into the right social circuit, corporate boardrooms and financial success. This was not to be. He was now faced with New York City schools. He quickly became bored, again skipped school and was finally dismissed. The friends he chose were drug users, yet I denied he was also using. My own life was full of problems — and for one entire summer, I vacillated between the extremes of suicide and eating disorders. Food was a drug I used to obliterate the pain.

We sought the help of family therapy. I learned that my protecting Pete was hurting him and keeping me from building a productive and healthy life on my own. Yet, I could not stop — if I didn't protect Pete and take responsibility for him, I would lose the only man I had in my life. Nothing was working. We fought constantly. His drug-induced behavior was responsible, I now know. At the time, however, unaware of his drug use, all I could see was that our life was crashing around us. I was powerless. It reached a crescendo when he hit me, and I called the police for the first of what would be many pleas for help. I was encouraged to go to family court and ask for an order of protection from Pete's abuse. Sitting in family court among members of other families with equally difficult situations was a humbling experience. The socio-economic lines became faint, as I finally recognized the depths to which Pete and I had sunk.

Our situation continued to deteriorate. We realized in family therapy that we had to separate — our lives were so entwined that neither of us could function. I had to let Pete go, so he could grow up. With neither job nor education, Pete found himself in a tough situation, but I stood my ground. He could not live in my home any longer. He moved out, found a job, and continued his stealing. The proceeds helped him buy the drugs that were now a continuation of his fantasyland. It is uncanny how it all played out from his early childhood. He was caught stealing from his job, and his only choice, so he thought, was to steal from me. One day I had let him spend the night at my apartment, whereupon he stole my bank card, and I finally had to come to terms with his crack addiction.

This time I could not deny it. I knew deep within me that he was the culprit. I was filled with the anguish only a parent can feel when forced to watch a child catapulting into the abyss of self-destruction. I was helpless to intervene.

From my bouts with bulimia, I knew of the Twelve-Step programs, and I made a frantic phone call. I went to a meeting. For the first time in my entire life, I was able to hear that I was not to blame. Somehow, just that much gave me the strength to go on. By some miracle, Pete agreed to go to a meeting, and then another miracle occurred. A place in a rehabilitation center opened up, and he went for treatment on his own accord. Slowly, painfully, and with much difficulty, we both began the long journey back to life. As part of his treatment, I was asked to participate in family week, and it was a painful, heartrending experience. All of my parental inadequacies were brought out in front of the group. I had to hear from Pete the deep pain he had suffered during the years when my business was my top priority. I learned how my father's alcoholism had influenced my life. My desire to succeed at any cost was a way for me to bolster my shattered sense of self. I also saw that my parents had not given me the foundation I needed to be a parent myself. I gradually realized I had done the best I could with what I had been given. Finally, I learned to forgive myself, and to give myself the opportunity to build a life on my own, separate from Pete.

I wish I could say it has been easy for the past two years, but I cannot do so. After his treatment, Pete still had to learn the hard way that life has responsibilities, and he lost several jobs in the process. He also had to learn the hard way to follow rules about paying rent and other bills. I had to learn to be firm with him. I would not allow him to live in my apartment if he did not work and contribute to the expenses. It was not easy coming home and finding him sleeping in the hallway of my building, because he had no other place to go. There were times when I was frightened that his depression would result in his committing suicide. I learned that he, like I, had a Higher Power, and Pete eventually found strength in the Twelve-Step programs. He began to build *his* life, not the one I wanted him to build. I do not agree with some of his life choices, but I support him unequivocally in his decision to choose sobriety as a way of life.

As I review the events of my life with Pete, I am grateful that he is my son. I see that we have been given a second chance. Being a mother has not been easy, and I am sure there will be trials in future years. After all, we are both human. I now consider our relationship pretty healthy. We are still close, yet free from the suffocation that results from a relationship built on need and fear.

Perhaps the most memorable symbol of our new, healthy life as mother and son lies in the culmination of one of my fondest dreams. Last year, I was married again, and Pete walked me down the aisle to meet the man who would become my husband, and then took his place among the other guests. I was finally free to embark on a new life of my own.

*   *   *

Christine illustrates how the web of self-blame can be complicated for parents of addicts. A spouse, however, can experience the same feelings of helplessness and desperation. Josephine shares her story as the spouse of a cocaine abuser.

* * *

JOSEPHINE

He was a happy-go-lucky kind of guy. He had everything going for him: good looks, sense of humor, money, bright future as an actor, little house by the sea, devoted dog, and people around him who loved him . . .

Yet when I first met him, it was something beyond all that which attracted me to him the most. There was an excitement about him, a sensation of living on the edge. I could never predict exactly what he was going to do next—he'd always surprise me, doing something silly or extreme which sometimes even caused himself harm. In those days I thought this intensity was "passion"; I now see it more as desperation.

We had immense fun together at the beginning. We'd stay up late at night over wine, a joint, maybe a bottle of Jack Daniels. It was very romantic and meaningful to me. We were in love. The reason he drank so much more than I did was because he was "a man," that's all. He could "handle" it.

Soon he began suggesting that we do coke once in a while. From once in a while it became every weekend. Before long, we were doing drugs of one kind or another pretty much all the time. He would give very convincing "reasons" why he always needed to get more. He "needed" drugs to get through an audition or job interview. He "needed" drugs to go over to his mother's house and deal with her craziness and her drinking (she was constantly drunk). He "needed" to get high to see this exciting new movie which just came out. He "deserved" to get high because he'd dealt with the IRS man this week. He "needed" drugs for good times, bad times, whatever times . . .

As time rolled on, I began to see the truth, which was that he hadn't worked as an actor for some time; almost a year, and his life was going downhill fast. He'd always talk about acting parts he almost got, and how his agent messed it up for him. He'd go on about "projects" he was working on which never really existed. He had a good front for the world, so good, in fact, that I'd bought into it myself. I wasn't doing much better with my own life, but it was taking as much energy as I had to deal with his problems. There was no time for my own.

I began to feel more and more resentful, that he wasn't really doing anything. I realize now that I had a poor self-image and very little self-confidence. By hooking up with him, and focusing everything on his life, I was trying to get an identity. Also, concentrating on his stuff was much less scary than taking a good look at my own life. I wasn't working; I kept thinking I'd get a job when things calmed down a bit. I was getting more and more depressed. Every day I'd wake up and see what kind of mood he was in. If he was in a good mood, my day went along fairly okay. If he was in a bad mood, my day would be dark, unbearable, and hopeless.

Once I began to see the extensiveness of his drug problem, I became more and more worried, but I continued to think I could handle it. I thought what he really needed was someone to love and support him like I knew I could, then he wouldn't need to do drugs anymore. I thought maybe I just wasn't trying hard enough, or maybe he was getting bored with me. There were also some days when he appeared to be very much in love with me and ecstatically happy.

Although I'd been using drugs along with him for a few months, I knew I had to stop, or it would really become a problem for me too. I was frightened of his reaction when I told him that I didn't want to do them anymore. Drugs were such a big part of his life. I was afraid he wouldn't want to be with me anymore. I slowly started using less, and, sure enough he'd get mad and accuse me of judging him, or being "no fun" anymore. It was a difficult decision for me to make. Part of me was becoming afraid of him. We started having terrible fights. I loved him and didn't want to lose him. However, no matter how hard I tried to convince him to cut down, he just went right on using.

If he wasn't high, he'd be so edgy and depressed that I'd be afraid to do or say anything that might "rub him the wrong way." I can see now what a prison I was living in. He'd usually find something to blow up at anyway, usually blaming me for whatever it was. The only way I knew how to deal with it was to lock my feelings up inside—my anger and disappointment. Every time he went off to get more drugs I felt betrayed. Sometimes when he was high he disgusted me and I didn't want him to come near me.

By this time his using had increased to the point where I was afraid he might overdose on something. I didn't know what to do. I knew he was lying to me about how much he bought. He'd do coke, then mix it with all kinds of other stuff. I felt afraid to go out in case he did too much of something. I couldn't tell my family what was going on because they would have just told me to leave him. I couldn't leave him! I loved him! Besides, who would be there to check up on him if I left? Who else would put up with all that? Anyway, I loved him. No one else could see his good side like I did. How can you abandon someone if you love them?

I spent every day trying to figure out how I could get him to stop using. He'd make promises to me, and break them within a few hours. I felt like our lives were being ruined. Here was everything I thought I wanted . . . and I was miserable. Part of me just wanted never to wake up again. I couldn't stand it.

One day, in the midst of one of his worst ever binges which had been going on for four days, I decided I'd had enough. I left the house early and went over to a girlfriend's house in tears. I told her everything. I was afraid he was going to overdose when he discovered I'd gone out. I just couldn't handle it anymore. She suggested I call his mother and ask her to go over to the house to check up on him. His mother went over there, slapped him around a bit to wake him up, cleaned up the house (he'd thrown Chinese food all over the kitchen walls in a rage the night before) and made him pull himself together for my return. Then she went home. When I got home that night he was still really high, stumbling around in an ugly, dazed stupor. I didn't know what he'd taken, but I knew it wasn't just cocaine. I hardly spoke to him, and planned to try to go to sleep and decide what to do in the morning.

We were awakened in the morning by a sudden telephone call from the local hospital. His mother was in intensive care. She had had an accident and was in critical condition. When we got there twenty minutes later, she was dead. She was fifty-eight years of age.

We'll never really know what happened to her. She apparently toppled off a chair in a restaurant and hit her head. Was it a stroke? A heart attack? No autopsy was done, so we'll never know. Back then, of course, I blamed myself: "Oh my God! It was too much for her to see her son strung out like that! It's all my fault! I should never have sent her over there that day." I have since understood that she was a woman suffering from high blood pressure who smoked two packs of cigarettes a day. She also drank at least a quart of vodka per day. She was an alcoholic. I've found out that my husband had a lot of "problem drinkers" in his family. Back then, I just thought I'd killed her.

Whatever the cause of her death, I was standing there in the hospital waiting room with my husband barely conscious, trying to grasp the news that his mother was lying there, dead, in the next room. I felt overwhelmed by the chaos of the situation, and by how desperately he needed me at that moment. I had reached the end. I had been planning to leave him. How could I now?

Pretty soon after that I went to see a counselor, because of my depression. I still felt responsible in some way for his mother's death. The counselor suggested I join a Twelve-Step program for family members, which I did, and gradually I began to feel better. It showed me that I had to take care of myself, that I was powerless over my husband's addiction. They helped me realize that my repeated attempts to get him into treatment were not working. I had to accept that seeking help for his addiction was going to have to be his own decision. I tried not to interfere, and eventually, through no effort of mine, he finally went into a detox unit, followed by a halfway house for addicts and alcoholics. I continued going to Twelve-Step meetings, and began to get back more of a sense of my own life. He had trouble staying sober for about a year, but then he finally started putting weeks and months together with no drugs or alcohol. We tried for another two years to work out the problems in our marriage, but finally we separated and then divorced.

Now, a few years later, I can look back and see how necessary it was for me to go through this whole experience. I had to learn that I cannot "rescue" another person from drug addiction. I've been able to see how plugged-in I was to his illness, and how I had no boundaries of my own. Without this experience, I probably would have gone through my whole life having one relationship after another with active alcoholics or drug abusers. I had a pattern of choosing people like him, with addictive tendencies. I don't know what it was in me that made me like that. Nevertheless, in my own recovery, I'm finding out that I can change that pattern. I can have relationships with healthy, sober people.

* * *

Jane offers another perspective as a parent whose child was addicted to cocaine and other drugs. Jane's story is a little different since she is an admitted recovering alcoholic and suffered through her daughter's addiction while recovering from her own.

* * *

JANE

The phone rang at 4:30 in the morning. It was my daughter, Jennifer, in San Francisco. "I'm on a street corner," she said with urgency and tension in her voice. "There's a cab driver who's been taking me all over to get away from those people. Mom, they're after me, where can I go, what can I do?" It was clear she was desperate, despondent and so wretched. Intellectually, I knew that I should let her reach her bottom and should not help her. On the other hand, she was my daughter. Intuitively, I put out my hand to her. "Do you want to come home? I'll get a ticket for you. What will you do for the rest of the night?" "The taxi driver will help me find a place," Jennifer said.

When she arrived at my apartment the next day, she was bedraggled. Her beautiful, silky, dark brown hair was matted and smelly, caked with dirt. She reeked of alcohol. Her eyes were bloodshot, her speech was hysterical. Her clothes were dirty. She was dirty. She had a rash and itched all over. As difficult as it was to touch her, I put my arms around her and was happy to have her because I loved her very much.

I had to let Jennifer go on her way. This was very important, yet difficult. I had been sober, myself, for seven years by this time. I had learned from my Twelve-Step program, that while I could put out my hand to her and care for her, I still had to let go. She stayed with me for a while, vanishing, returning; I didn't know what she was doing but I knew she was getting worse. I prayed for the knowledge of my Higher Power's will for me and for Jennifer. I went to Twelve-Step self help meetings for family members and was given wonderful support.

Jennifer found a job with a fellow who was very ill and needed someone to look after him. Later, I was to find out that he was a cocaine dealer. He was suffering from a fatal illness from which he later died. Jennifer moved in with him.

I went to the West Coast to spend Christmas with my other daughter. Jennifer went to the town in Connecticut where she was born, to visit with her old friends. I knew they were all drinking and using drugs and I was not happy because it was a very bad situation. Once again I had to let go. When I phoned her there, her friends told me that even by their standards, Jennifer's behavior was bizarre. What exactly happened when she was there, I don't really know. She kept calling me in California, sounding hysterical and not making any sense. Her sister and I agreed that Jennifer was very, very ill and there wasn't anything we could do about it. We could only allow her to be sick without interfering. Let her go and let her do what she had to do.

Jennifer called and said she had come back to New York by train. Apparently, on the train, something had happened to her that was truly peculiar. It was never clear to me exactly what had happened, she just said there was some big problem with the train. It hit me that she could have been close to death. Her disease was killing her and it was killing me, too, but I couldn't do anything about it. That was the most important part for me to understand and accept. There was nothing I could do.

Acceptance finally came to me at this point and with it some serenity, although it was still a very painful time. I think of the episode of the train ride and my other daughter as the catalysts. All I could do was let her know that I loved her. I was there for her, and I didn't condemn her for using.

On my return from California, I began going to many meetings of a Twelve-Step family program for family members. I knew this

would help me. It was also one more thing I could do for Jennifer
. . . take care of myself.

On January 15, I was sitting in my office when I got a phone call
from Jennifer, who was sobbing hysterically. She didn't know
where she was, only that she was in a friend's apartment some-
where. She had lost her bag and coat. She had been mixed up in
something at an after hours club the night before and there had been
some kind of shooting. I asked her if she wanted some help and she
answered that she did. I said, "Take a cab and I will meet you." I
called someone I knew at a rehabilitation hospital and asked if they
could admit her to detox. They said yes. They said if she did want
to go to the hospital they could take her. There was one bed available.

Jennifer arrived in a taxi, shouting at the driver at the top of her
lungs. Her hair was matted and stringy. It was freezing cold. When
I paid the taxi driver, he looked at me and said, "Lady, I don't
know what's the matter with her, but she's a sick cookie and she's
nuts!" He shook his head.

She was very upset but not hysterical. "Do you want to go to a
hospital?" I asked her. "Do they have a bed?" she asked. "Yes,
they have a bed." With that I rang up the hospital and they said to
bring her right along.

What she meant about the hospital bed was that she wanted to
sleep because she was exhausted. She wasn't even thinking about
treatment. For me what a bed meant was treatment. We discovered
our different interpretations many years later. She was insured on
my insurance policy, a small blessing. So all the paper work was
taken care of and she was admitted.

What an enormous relief it was for me to have her in the hospital.
In recalling the time when I first thought that perhaps there was a
chance for recovery if she wanted it, I still shake and tremble. Tears
come to my eyes. Because I got sober without a rehab, I knew how
important they had become and what a head start they gave to alcoholics and drug abusers. It was natural that I wanted her to stay in
the rehab for twenty-eight days. However, after five days in the
detox, Jennifer went home and began attending Twelve-Step meetings. I stayed in touch with her, but again I had to let her go, had to
let her work her recovery herself. I could not jump in and tell her

what to do. I found it very hard not to direct her sobriety; mothers have always taught their daughters, and pulling back on this was tough.

Her sobriety has been a miracle to me. It's again January and her anniversary has just passed. She has a beautiful sobriety of which I am exceptionally proud. We have had our "ups and downs" in the years she has been sober. At times it has not been easy. Having a sober daughter, however, rather than a dead daughter, is worth all the pain I went through.

I think the turning point came for me when I finally accepted that I could do nothing about her disease even if she were to die. Once I had this realization, I was able to continue living my life. Better still, two weeks later, she called for help. This is a powerful message for me.

*   *   *

Finally, Alex tells his story as the husband of a cocaine addict. He too, expresses many of the same feelings.

*   *   *

ALEX

I thought she was everything I needed and wanted. She was beautiful, warm, intelligent, funny. And, she liked to drink. She loved champagne. The first time I opened her refrigerator I found nothing but three bottles of champagne and some water. She explained that she was on a diet and didn't want much food around. I also noticed how filthy her kitchen was. So I decided to clean it for her. Later, I took on the role of always cleaning up after my wife.

Drugs and alcohol were always present in our marriage. I thought it was mostly a waste of time, but she said it was just recreational and a fun thing to share. I wanted to please her so I did it a few times myself and soon drugs were a part of every social occasion. She loved it. She began consuming larger amounts than I thought were "normal." It was happening a lot more frequently than I was willing to admit. I now see that my denial was already well in place.

I was getting fed up. We began to argue. Her excuse was that drugs were OK unless they became a problem. She saw no problem. Her friends were also using, especially cocaine. They justified their behavior by saying that cocaine was not addictive.

I began to feel that my wife really wasn't there for me. She was either angry, high or impatient. She'd yell and scream for no reason. I started having affairs which became a problem when my wife found out. We had horrible fights followed by more drinking and drugging, then guilt, pain and craziness. Things got worse. I changed jobs frequently. A freelance photographer, my earnings were unreliable. The drinking and drugging went on, and my infidelities increased.

Four years into the marriage we hit our first "bottom." My wife decided she had had enough. I came home one day and she was gone. I found out that she had moved in with an old boyfriend. I persuaded her to come back. We tried to work things out but it didn't last. When she ran off to her parents' house they sent her back. She had started stealing from them and drinking heavily in their house.

We tried again. I said that perhaps she had a drinking problem. I offered to get help myself. I still wanted to work it out. She'd say she'd stop, then a few days later it would start all over again. The cycle seemed endless. Our Soho loft became a haven for drug addicts and wild parties. I was unable to stop them. Our fights had become increasingly violent. There were knives, broken bottles and sometimes she'd get hysterical.

I thought I could control her drugging forcibly. I'd hit and yell. I threatened her with hospital and police. She was stealing from me — some of my equipment was missing. She'd disappear at night: "Honey, I'm going to the store to get you a sandwich," and she would disappear until 6 o'clock the next morning. Her personality would change, particularly when she used cocaine. At first she'd be talkative and nice, then as the evening wore on, she'd become progressively more distant, belligerent and hostile.

The flip side of my violent behavior was my remorse and desire to please her. I bought her expensive gifts. I took her out to dinner. Nothing, however, changed her behavior. I pleaded, I begged. At one point I even bought her drugs thinking that would at least keep her home. When I wouldn't do cocaine with her she'd say we were incompatible. If I did drugs with her I felt bad about myself.

One weekend she disappeared for two days. When she finally came home, she was bruised and battered, wearing only one shoe. She was crying. She smelled of alcohol and sweat and looked like she'd been crawling through a sewer. She was disgusting. She said she'd been in a fight with one of our friends, and he'd beaten her up. I felt sorry for her, but at the same time I was angry. I didn't know what to do.

I brought her into the house. I washed her, took care of her clothes, fed her. She said I should go and beat up this man to avenge her honor. She was really pressuring me. So I went to see him. They'd been drinking and drugging. His drug of choice was freebase. My need to please her was still so great that when I got home I told her I'd seen him, had a big fight, and avenged her honor. Soon she disappeared again for three days. After a few more similar occasions, I finally told her she had to leave.

This was a big change because I had always been the one to rescue her. This time I couldn't take it anymore. She moved in with some friends, and I sublet another apartment. Sometimes she'd come and stay with me, and just sleep. After another disappearing act, I went to her apartment and forced my way in. When I got inside, I was horrified. The place was a pig sty. Drug paraphernalia was everywhere. Clothes strewn about. There was even dog excrement on the floor.

I was scared. I called some friends and arranged to move her things out. As we were packing, my wife walked in. She began yelling and screaming at me. I pleaded with her to let me help her. She looked different. She'd lost a lot of weight and was obviously undernourished. It was a very, very sad moment for me. She insisted that I leave, so I did.

Two friends and I armed with .357 Magnums staked out her house. We were going to force her into a hospital. What I was doing was truly insane. She had disappeared again. Finally I contacted the police and filed a missing person complaint. When I went to the police station, a detective took me aside and confided in me that he'd been through a similar experience. He explained that he'd done all kinds of illegal things himself to try to get his wife to stop doing cocaine and drinking. If he had tried everything he knew to stop his wife, what made me think that I'd be able to succeed with mine?

He also explained to me that maybe I had a problem. I was so involved in her life that I was willing to put my *own life* in danger to protect hers. He suggested that I go to Co-Anon, saying it was a program for friends and families of drug addicts. All he said was "It helps people, it works." I kept telling him I did not have a problem. My *wife* was the one with the problem. I described to him all the things I'd been through. He said he had been through the same thing, and that this program works. It sounded too easy. Too much like religion. I thought about it overnight, and I went to a meeting.

What I heard was not what I wanted to hear. I wanted to know how to stop her drugging, how to help her and how to save my marriage. Instead, what I heard was stories similar to mine, with the difference that their lives had changed and improved. They just kept telling me to come back to more meetings. They gave me literature to read and a schedule of meetings.

Strangely enough, things started to change. My rescue mission with my wife started to look different to me. I saw how my own behavior had become totally irrational. I began to consider what was important to me. This happened over a period of months. It did not happen overnight. It became easier as time went by. I was spending more time in the Co-Anon rooms, developing new friendships, reading the literature, trying to understand what the program was about. It became a way of life for me, a way to keep the focus on myself. I began to look at myself in an honest way for the first time. I'd spent most of my life focused on other people, judging them.

Her family finally got involved in the program in another city. I came to understand what my role had been in all this madness. Essentially, I was given my life back.

* * *

A cocaine addict can cause as much trouble to an employer as to a relative, although trouble of a different sort. Some employers, especially in small businesses, may be forced to rely on the cocaine addict's skills to stay afloat. Employers can also find themselves in the position of repeatedly lending money, or "advances" to an employee who might have a cocaine problem. This can be very difficult to handle, especially when the employee has been with the company for a while. All too easily, allowances can be made for poor job performance, or the employer may realize he or she is being lied to, but not know how to confront the employee. Sometimes the whole business may suffer as a result.

Similarly, although it may be difficult to work for a demanding boss, it is close to impossible to work for someone who is addicted to cocaine. An employer on coke can make irrational decisions which may affect the livelihood of all employees. According to his or her mood swings, the boss may also subject employees to unwarranted abusive behavior. A cocaine addict's behavior will often be unpredictable and having an unpredictable boss can be nerve-racking.

Cocaine addiction can, in fact, have a profound effect on anybody who interacts with the addict. By the time an individual's use of cocaine becomes addictive, a number of other people have usually been affected. Watching an addict destroy him or herself with cocaine can be devastating to the onlooker's own physical, emotional and mental health. Most often, because so much focus is being placed on the addicted person, the onlookers and loved ones can be unaware of the stress they themselves are undergoing.

THE SPECIAL DANGERS OF COCAINE ADDICTION

Although the dynamics of addiction may be similar for all drugs, cocaine addiction can often be particularly devastating on a family. Cocaine is highly addictive and therefore the effects can be felt by the family very quickly. One can become addicted to cocaine in a few months. Before long, sizable sums of family money—funds put aside for special occasions, personal savings—may disappear, as may household valuables. Often seeming to occur out of the blue, this brings home the danger of addiction.

Sometimes a person can become addicted to cocaine with no previous experience of heavy drinking, no earlier use of other drugs, no sign of addictive tendencies. Does this mean that once the co-caine addict makes the decision to simply stay away from cocaine, he or she will be all right? Possibly. In most cases, however, if a problem with cocaine has already developed, there will always be a danger of abusing other substances.

In order to avoid the pitfall of "switching addictions," most treatment programs recommend total abstinence from all drugs (in-cluding alcohol). This treatment philosophy seems to have a much greater success rate than others which might allow the use of, say, alcohol or marijuana. Although many cocaine addicts complain ve-hemently about having to give up alcohol and other drugs in order to recover from cocaine addiction, it has been shown repeatedly that an addict becomes much more vulnerable to picking up cocaine again if he or she drinks alcohol or takes other mind-altering sub-stances. This is because once under the influence of the other drug, their judgement is impaired, and their resistance to the urge to pick up cocaine is lowered.

If the family or close friends of the addict are uneducated in this regard, they can unknowingly perpetuate the addiction by offering the addict alcohol or some other drug. Some addicts complain that their job or profession "requires" them to use cocaine in order to be accepted by their colleagues. It is important to remember that co-caine addiction is a potentially fatal disease. It gets worse, not bet-ter. The addict may have to decide to give up the "cocaine life-style" along with the cocaine; not to could mean losing *everything*. The family's support is vital in this decision, not just in supporting the addict's abstinence from drugs and alcohol, but also in creating a drug-free home.

If the addict continues to drink or use other drugs, he or she is avoiding the experience of life on life's terms. Family members can unintentionally sabotage the addict's recovery by continuing to use other drugs in front of the addict.

The fact that cocaine is illegal has a subtle and profound effect on the family or anyone who is closely connected to the addict. It means that anyone who knows that the addict is using cocaine must collude in illegal behavior. There is a constant underlying threat of being found out by the police. The implications of arrest, convic-tion and possible jail are frightening for the family, and the consequences can be devastating and humiliating. Buying cocaine often involves going to "dealers" or buying from strangers in the street. An addict can never be sure he or she will avoid police "busts" or frames. Many addicts "deal" themselves, and the family often lives in a state of constant paranoia about late night phone calls, knocks on the door or visits from sometimes desperate individuals.

Cocaine is expensive, so large sums of money exchange hands, sometimes putting the family in potentially volatile situations involving crime and weapons. A child growing up in this kind of atmosphere will undoubtedly suffer psychological consequences. The drastic mood changes ("cravings," "highs," and "crashes") which accompany cocaine use are confusing and deeply disturbing for children.

Some cocaine abusers can go for many months without even touching the drug, rationalizing that therefore they don't have a "problem." They can sometimes resume a normal lifestyle, swear that this is "the last time that they'll ever touch cocaine," and then, for no apparent reason, start using again. This is called "periodic" substance abuse. The cycle of addiction continues as if the addict had never stopped, getting progressively worse and more destructive each time. This can be particularly devastating for family members, because each time the addict stops, they think their lives have been restored to normal, and each time he or she starts again, the disappointment and anger take a greater toll.

How many family members have lived in dread of the day their loved one comes home stoned? How many spouses have kept dinner warm for their husband or wife, only to finally get that phone call, with the familiar tone of voice, telling them "something came up" and he or she won't be coming home.

These experiences can be so agonizing, that members of the addict's family sometimes get very caught up in "detective" work: trying to figure out whether the addict is using or not, and if so, how much. They find themselves listening to the addict's phone conversations, searching his or her clothing or belongings, checking up on his or her whereabouts, or following the addict to track his or her movements. This behavior can soon develop into obsession, and can seriously damage the family member's own mental health. Although people do this with good intentions (to try to save the addict), it does nothing to help the addict and, in fact, often antagonizes him or her. If this behavior continues, the family member can become so obsessed that he or she totally neglects his or her own life.

SOME COMMON RESPONSES TO THE ADDICT

Cocaine addiction works fast. As soon as the symptoms start to show themselves, they create tension in the family. Resentments build up. Tempers begin to flare. Whether the family knows about cocaine abuse or not, there may be increasing arguments and fights, and the cocaine abuser may start having "crashes" during which he or she is irritable, depressed and even paranoid.

Family members often get exasperated by the addict's changes in mood and behavior. It is very difficult not to take it personally when someone you love is extremely volatile and unpredictable. Family members often start behaving erratically themselves, reacting to the tension and uneasiness in the home, or simply resenting the addict's continued use of cocaine. Marital problems can result and children will inevitably feel the backlash. Frequently, children develop difficulties in school when there is an addiction problem at home. They may start cutting classes or getting behind in school work. It has been known for some children to develop concentration problems or even learning disabilities. Whatever the manifestation, it is unwise to underestimate the consequences children may experience resulting from an addiction problem at home. As with use of any mind-altering chemical, there is an increased risk of physical or sexual abuse in the family.

If a family member suspects that there is a drug problem, their reactions of suspicion, distrust, hurt or fear tend to lead to worry and depression. If they *know* there is a drug problem, their deep feelings of frustration, anger, helplessness and loneliness can be overwhelming. We have seen family members who *know* there is a problem respond in a variety of ways:

Some people try to deal with the problem by "joining" the addict. They use cocaine with the addict, hoping to decrease the cocaine supply so that the addict will run out. This rarely succeeds; the addict will usually find more cocaine if he or she wants to, regardless of how much is left. Others use cocaine with the addict because they are afraid if they don't, the addict won't want to spend time with them. Still others use with the addict in order to keep an eye on how much he or she is using. Then there are those who are simply well on their way to becoming addicted themselves, or already have a problem.

Other family members try to deal with the addiction through strict discipline and punishment. A firm approach may be beneficial, but a punitive attitude almost always backfires. Our clinical experience has revealed that a strong disciplinary approach does little to help the addict reach a voluntary decision to give up cocaine. It must be his or her *own* decision. If they are being forced, or punished, they might easily react with defiance and continue to do even more cocaine. If an addict threatens to do more cocaine, or leave, the family member should be careful not to become intimidated by this. Allowing the addict to blackmail you is not beneficial to the addict. If the addict is given the power to intimidate simply by making the threats, the family members are setting themselves up for being "walked all over."

Family members should not be reluctant to set their own limits. It can be helpful to establish clear boundaries with the addict about what is *acceptable* and what is *unacceptable* behavior. Each family needs to assess what they are *not* willing to tolerate, and find where to draw the line. A decision to no longer give the addict money can be very helpful if the money has just been going toward buying drugs (which it frequently does). It is a good idea to establish certain family "ground rules" that the addict and everyone else must follow if they are to continue living in the house. The importance of setting boundaries is to minimize the victimization of family members. (These issues are more fully addressed later in this chapter.)

If family members suffer every week, for example, because the family paycheck goes toward buying cocaine, some system is necessary for placing the money in the bank and keeping it there. If the addict has violent outbursts, the family must set themselves a "bottom line" of what they are willing to tolerate, and be prepared to leave or call the police if necessary. Idle threats are ineffectual; the addict will see through them. They must know that you mean business, that you'll follow through on whatever ground rules you set up, including asking the addict to leave. If this is the case, it is suggested that you obtain support (family, friends, self-help groups and/or counseling) in order to carry through with this decision.

Fear of verbal or physical abuse may sometimes keep family members from confronting the addict. If we allow the addict to intimidate us, we too become prisoners of cocaine. Family members are frequently too frightened to tell anyone else about the problem; the longer the addiction is kept secret, the more difficult it is to expose it.

Family members who keep the addict's behaviors secret join in a "conspiracy of silence," one that forces the family into isolation. Because they often feel ashamed of what's going on in their home, they stop socializing with friends and cut back on social activities. The family then suffers from a feeling of alienation and separation from the rest of society. The longer the family carries this burden, the more difficult it is to break out of the isolation. The stigma attached to cocaine addiction makes it more difficult to seek help when you think the community will reject you for having an addicted family member. Despite progress in the field of alcoholism and addiction, society still views addiction as a "moral weakness" rather than an illness. People associated with an addict sometimes fear that if the addiction problem is revealed, it may jeopardize their chances for employment, cause their children to be ridiculed at school, their neighbors to gossip about them, their families to ostracize them or society to simply label them "weak" or "sick" for loving a drug addict. Some of these fears may be realistic, but *none* of them should prevent family members from facing the truth and seeking help.

It is important to remember that a common pattern in addiction is for the addict to blame the family members for all of his or her problems, using rationalizations such as: "Who wouldn't use cocaine with a wife like you at home?" or "It's the pressure around here that's making me do coke!" or "How else do you expect me to relax when you're nagging me all the time!" The addict might feel, internally, out of control with his or her own life and addiction and this is such a painful realization that most addicts protect themselves by unconsciously blaming others around them. No one wants to admit to an addiction problem; most people will blame *anyone* or *anything* else rather than admit that they themselves have a problem! Family members should keep this in mind when the addict is criticizing them, and be careful not to "take on" unnecessary blame.

It is enormously difficult not to nag, plead or complain to the addict when the drug use is having a destructive impact on the family. Nagging can often exacerbate the situation, however, because it gives the addict yet another "excuse" to get high. The nagging irritates the addict, causing him or her to feel justified to use more cocaine; the family member nags and complains even *more*, and the addict then has the perfect "excuse" to use even *more*. This cycle can continue for a long time, both parties caught in a "revolving door" with no way out.

It is helpful for family members to remember the following about addiction:

YOU DIDN'T CAUSE IT
YOU CAN'T CONTROL IT
YOU CAN'T CURE IT

This slogan is known as the "Three C's" in family Twelve-Step programs. The "Three C's" reinforce the concept that addiction is a disease, and that nothing anyone does will help the addict to stop using unless the addict wants to stop for him or herself. The "Three C's" also addresses the guilt that many family members (particularly parents) experience in the face of addiction. Family members often ask professionals whether the addiction is their fault. They somehow feel responsible for the addiction and unduly punish themselves for it. They worry that it was something they did or didn't do when the addict was growing up. Spouses often feel that perhaps they haven't shown the addict enough love, or just the opposite, that they've smothered the addict. Few family members are spared from this kind of self-torture.

There is usually a constellation of reasons causing addiction: psychological, physiological, social, environmental and circumstantial. IT IS A WASTE OF TIME TO BLAME ONESELF FOR THE ADDICTION. IT IS NO ONE PERSON'S FAULT. In the process of treatment, or in self-help groups, family members sometimes do evaluate their *own* behavior in relation to the addict, discovering things about themselves that they want to change. There may be occasions when one regrets something said, or the one time one let the addict down in some way . . . We are all human; no one is perfect. Certainly everyone makes mistakes, but the past is *over* and there's no point in going over it and punishing oneself. The most helpful approach is to simply begin with what one *has*, and make the best of it, whether that includes seeking professional help, or finding a self-help group in order to work through these feelings. Remember, regardless of what happened in the past, most likely no one *forced* cocaine up the addict's nose. Even if a family member feels that he or she helped initiate the addict into using cocaine, the addict made the decision to continue to use cocaine, and must make the decision to stop.

"ENABLING" AND "CODEPENDENCY"

What really happens to the family when one member becomes addicted to cocaine? Once one realizes a loved one is in trouble, the family member's first instinct is usually to want to help. He or she wants to do *anything* possible to fix the problem so the loved one doesn't have to suffer. This is, of course, a normal reaction for any family member.

When dealing with addiction, however, one is no longer dealing with a normal situation. "Helping" can often be the *least* productive thing one can do; it can even make the situation worse.

A family member may not want to hear this; he or she may well be thinking at this point: "What *else* are you supposed to do, stand back and watch them suffer?"

After trying everything one can do to help the situation, the last thing one may want to hear is that *this* in *itself* could be detrimental. That's too exasperating; it could make one feel like giving up. It is never *wrong* to have the desire to help someone. The problem is in that as long as the addict is "helped" out of each uncomfortable situation, he or she will never learn why he or she got there in the first place! The following is typical: "Jerry" continually places himself in debt buying drugs. Each time he runs out of money, someone (usually his mother, his sister or his best friend) "helps" him pay off the debt; thus, Jerry is forever protected from the uncomfortable consequences of owing his dealers money or having his electricity switched off. How will he fully understand what it feels like to have spent all his money on drugs unless he actually has *no more money?* The best thing in the world for Jerry might be to experience a week or two with no electricity.

Regardless of how uncomfortable it may be to imagine standing back and watching the person you love suffer, the agony of prolonged addiction is far worse. If the addiction continues, it is potentially far more dangerous than living for a few weeks without electricity, or even losing a job. Whatever it takes to get the addict's attention is exactly what needs to occur as a consequence of his or her own drug use. An addict can never feel the "pinch" of his or her behavior if people are always there to "cover" for him or her. He or she will never suffer the natural outcome. If someone is always there to "make it better," how can the addict realize how chaotic his or her life has really become? If the problem is continually "fixed," everything will just feel fine again for the addict, and he or she will repeat the same behavior. What incentive is there to change?

In short, the problem with "helping" is that it PROTECTS THE ADDICT FROM FACING THE CONSEQUENCES OF HIS OR HER OWN BEHAVIOR. He or she will have no motivation to obtain help. If family members and friends continue to help get the addict out of trouble, they are not, in fact, helping the addict—they are doing what's called "ENABLING" the addict to continue.

There are many different forms of enabling behavior. Whatever the cause of the addiction, it is a fact that the family's interaction and the immediate environment of the addict make a big difference. Family members, work associates and friends of the addict have a responsibility to learn to identify and stop their *own* "enabling" behavior toward the addict.

To help identify whether you may be "enabling" the addicted person in your life, answer the questions on the following check list as honestly as you can:

ENABLING CHECKLIST

1. Have you ever covered a financial debt for the addict?
2. Have you ever made a phone call to cancel an appointment on the addict's behalf?
3. Have you ever "called in sick" or made excuses for the addict to his or her job or school?

4. Have you ever permitted the addict to get physically abusive and failed to call the police?
5. Have you let the addict come and live with you because he or she has "run out of money?"
6. Have you repeatedly loaned the addict money?
7. Have you ever bailed the addict out of jail for an arrest connected with drug abuse?
8. Have you ever excused the addict from keeping a commitment because he or she is "depressed?"
9. Are you afraid to confront the addict about his or her use of drugs for fear of violence?
10. Are you afraid to confront the addict about his or her use of drugs for fear that he or she will leave you?
11. Do you sometimes think the drug use is not so bad because at least he or she is only using *at home?*
12. Do you sometimes act as if you believe the addict's excuses even when you know he or she is lying?
13. Do you sometimes think it's because of *you* that the addict got high?
14. Do you prefer not to talk to anyone about the problem because you're ashamed?
15. Do you let the addict come back in the house even after he or she has been physically destructive?
16. Do you make excuses to your children for the addict's drug-induced behavior(s)?
17. Do you pretend that the addict is "sick" when really he or she is coming off a cocaine binge?
18. Have you ever taken drugs with the addict so you can be together?
19. Have you ever obtained drugs for the addict?
20. Do you threaten to leave the addict, and then not follow through on leaving?

If you answered yes to three or more of these questions, you have probably been "enabling" someone in your life to continue using drugs. Although your intentions have no doubt been the best, if you want your loved one to stop using drugs, *your role* in this is to stop "enabling" now.

DENIAL

As you've already seen, "denial" is one of the hallmarks of addiction. Just as the addict may be denying to him or herself how much cocaine he or she is using, so family members can deny the severity of the addiction and how much it affects them. Denial is an unconscious mechanism with which the mind protects itself from an uncomfortable truth. When an addict looks you straight in the eye and informs you that there is no problem, it can be all too easy to believe it despite your concern. After all, they should know, shouldn't they? The last thing family members and friends of drug abusers want to believe is that their loved one is addicted. They would much rather believe it's a "phase" he or she is going through, or that "this time" he or she will be able to stop. Family and friends want to believe the addict has it under control. The problem is, each time the addict promises to stop and doesn't, the failure becomes more damaging to the family member.

Because this is so painful, family members and close friends of addicts may minimize the severity of the drug abuse. They may tell themselves: "It's not really so bad"; "everyone does it"; "he only uses on weekends"; or "it can't be so bad, she hasn't lost her job yet." This can go on for a long time until they finally accept that cocaine is controlling their loved one, not the other way around.

Family members may also start to question their own perceptions. If you sense something is going on, but it is constantly denied, you may soon end up doubting *yourself*. This self-doubt is extremely damaging, since it means you are disconnected from your own warning signals. You may soon start to doubt yourself in other areas too—in fact, you may eventually run the risk of losing the ability to trust your own instincts entirely.

CO-DEPENDENCY*

This loss of selfhood is sometimes referred to in the field of chemical dependency as "co-dependency." Co-dependency de-

---

*This word has become widely exploited and almost clichéd in the field of addiction.

velops when someone focuses so much on taking care of another person's needs, that they ignore their own. Co-dependents expend so much energy and time thinking about other people's problems or behavior, that their own emotional, physical, mental and spiritual needs are seriously neglected.

A co-dependent may often feel that another person's needs are greater than his or her own. He or she will often choose to be with people whose problems appear to be more serious than their own, thus necessitating a form of submission and self-sacrifice. On the surface these intentions seem honorable and worthy of praise; our society condones these values and they are heralded by the media, organized religion, education, government and the helping professions. There is nothing wrong with the principle of wanting to help someone, but if it results in suffering and dysfunction on the part of the helping person, it means they have depleted their own inner resources too much in order to be of assistance to others.

By focusing on another person, co-dependents often neglect their own development to the detriment of their own career and self-esteem. They may sometimes believe that if they can just satisfy the other person, then the other person will be able to satisfy them. In believing this, they are placing their happiness in someone else's hands, and looking outside themselves for fulfillment. This may bring temporary relief (as does using drugs, drinking or any other addictive behavior), but eventually their own inner depletion will catch up with them. The person in whom they've placed their happiness will inevitably let them down, (being human and fallible), just as the drugs or alcohol will eventually stop working for the addict. A co-dependent may gradually get caught up in trying to meet someone else's needs, just as an addict can become involved in the progression of his or her addiction. In this sense, co-dependency is, in itself, an addiction.

A family member or close friend of an addict may very easily become obsessed with controlling the quantity the addict uses. The motive is to help the addict, but the result is that the co-dependent loses his or her own inner balance in the process. It is only a matter of time before the co-dependent may begin to feel taken advantage of and victimized. Some co-dependents may continue in this cycle for many years. They may feel self-righteous and even superior to the addict, thinking at least they are maintaining some kind of equilibrium, compared to the more obvious disarray of the addict's circumstances.

They may, indeed, be carrying a large proportion of the addict's responsibilities, but it is the distortion of the illness which makes them believe they are somehow superior. What they don't realize is that they are locked inside the same prison of obsession, disappointment and lack of fulfillment as the addict. They may blame the addict for their unhappiness, but the longer they focus on the addict's problems and neglect their own, the longer they choose to continue living in their version of the same agony. They may feel superior, but they are often just as unhappy as the addict. The theme of co-dependency is the illusion of power through self-sacrifice.

The effects of co-dependency can manifest themselves as physical illness, depression, anxiety, stress and/or emotional numbness. There is often a pervasive feeling of being out of control, which leads to an overpowering need to control more. The more the co-dependent tries to control the addict or other people around him or her, the more frustrated he or she will become. The fact is, no one has control over anyone else. The co-dependent will sometimes go to ridiculous lengths to try to regulate the behavior of an addict. For example, Bill, a young man from New York, handcuffed his girlfriend to the stairwell in order to prevent her from buying more cocaine—of course, as soon as he released her, she went out and did just that. Children growing up in a household where one parent is addicted to drugs or alcohol, frequently report in treatment that the parent exhibiting the most "crazy" behavior is not the substance abuser, but the spouse!

The only way out for co-dependents is to start putting the focus back on their own needs, their own lives. Co-dependents can begin to help themselves by:

1. Seeking out and regularly attending a self-help group for families and friends of addicts, or co-dependents.
2. Attending group therapy (specific for co-dependence), and/or seeking individual counseling/psychotherapy.
3. Attending educational series on co-dependency and addiction in hospitals and drug rehabilitation centers.

4. Building an ongoing support system from self-help groups, therapy groups and trusted friends to help make and sustain the changes in behavior necessary to break the patterns of enabling and co-dependency.

HOW TO AVOID CO-DEPENDENT
OR ENABLING BEHAVIOR

Avoid Taking Too Much Responsibility

When you feel an impulse to take care of something for the addict, stop and think. Ask yourself if what you're about to do is really your responsibility, or is it the addict's? Is that bill you're about to pay really yours? Is it actually *your* responsibility to call his boss and explain why he's late? Is it your job to buy gifts for her relatives so they won't know she's forgotten again?

Whatever the task is, if the responsibility is returned to its rightful owner — the addict — you will be doing both of you a favor in the long run. Keep in mind, however, that when you give back the responsibility to the addict, there is no guarantee he or she will do the thing you want him or her to do. Therefore, it is wise to plan an alternative for yourself. Either have an alternative action in mind, or do the thing yourself if you have absolutely no choice and your own well-being is at stake. An example of this is if you're living with the addict and he or she has not fulfilled his or her obligation to pay the electricity bill, the choice is either to pay the bill or have your electricity turned off. The discomfort caused to you by losing the service may be greater than the discomfort caused by the addict's neglect of his or her responsibility.

Set Boundaries

Get support and professional help to decide what is acceptable and what is unacceptable behavior on the part of the addict. Physical abuse is an example of unacceptable behavior that can never be tolerated. Each situation is different and each household must come up with its own specific guidelines and boundaries. But remember, whatever you decide, be prepared to follow through with firm action; that can mean confiscating keys or money, leaving the house, even calling the police. The addict will soon find out whether you are bluffing. Joe, the parent of one addict, reports that he tolerated years of having his money and credit cards stolen before one night he threw his son out of the house and changed the locks. He said this was probably the most painful thing he's ever had to do; he spent the night wondering if the boy had been murdered or died of an overdose. Instead, soon afterward, his son decided to ask for help and entered a drug rehabilitation center. Firm action sometimes offers the best chance of making an addict face up to the reality of his or her situation.

Don't Protect the Addict

When an addict's drug use starts to cause problems socially, physically, professionally, psychologically or emotionally, it is wise to not protect him or her from the results. Don't minimize the problem, and don't "enable" the addict in any way. Don't agree to keep secrets from other family members or friends, don't smooth things over, don't cover for the addict financially. Most importantly, don't let the addict manipulate you into doing things for him or her. (See Enabling Checklist for further examples.)

Tell the addict: "I'm sorry, I can't do that for you," or "You're going to have to do that for yourself, it's not my responsibility," or "I love you, but I'm not prepared to help you unless you get help for yourself first."

Stay Out of the Addict's Treatment/Recovery

Before an addict is ready to get help there is little anyone can do to persuade them. Rather than ignoring that it exists, however, you can let the addict know that you think there's a drug problem and that it seriously concerns you and affects your life. You can say that you'd like to help, but that you know the addict must overcome the problem for him or herself.

Once the addict is in some kind of recovery program, family members and friends are often tempted to get involved with the treatment. It is just as important that you stay out of the addict's recovery as it is that he or she enters treatment on his or her own initiative. Addicts have to do this for *themselves*. If you constantly ask questions, give opinions, go to their recovery meetings with them or telephone their therapist/counselor, you are once more taking away the addict's initiative and responsibility. This can seriously jeopardize treatment, unless it is a planned, integral part of the treatment program.

Never call and cancel the addict's counseling sessions, or any other of his or her appointments. Let the addict make those phone calls and let the addict seek and receive help without you.

There can be other problems as well. Some family members find themselves resenting the addict's recovery "program" friends, or being jealous of his or her new social outlets. If you feel angry that the addict spends so much time in self-help meetings or therapy sessions, find some of your *own* to go to or occupy yourself with friends and hobbies.

Michelle, the wife of an addict for seven years, says that when her husband found Cocaine Anonymous he spent as much time away from home as when he'd been using! She was angry at the people in his recovery group who treated him like a hero because he had ninety days clean and sober. They didn't know what *she'd* been through with his coke habit, and *she* was still the one at home doing all the work!

It is simply unwise to expect too much from the recovering addict in early sobriety. He or she faces a long and slow transformation, and great patience is required on the part of family members. The best results are found when the family lets the addict know of their love and firm support in recovery, but they leave the recovery up to him or her.

Seeking Help

Family members may know they need help, but may not have a clue as to what kind of help, or where to find it. We will outline here some of the alternatives. Before that, however, it is important to understand the difference between help for the family members and help for the addict.

Family members usually seek help to find a way to stop the addict from using cocaine. However, if the addict refuses to seek help with them, they often feel there's no point in continuing treatment for themselves. There are two things to consider here: (1) help for the addict, (2) help for the family members *themselves*.

It is true that no one can stop an addict from using cocaine unless he or she decides to stop; the addict must "hit bottom" and make his or her own decision. Sometimes, this means the family must stop their own enabling and co-dependent behavior. If the family gets treatment or support from a self-help organization for *themselves*, the chances are that they will start handling the addict with more appropriate and educated responses. The chain of events in the family system indicates that although the addict may not like it at first, in the long run, this change in behavior is often what motivates him or her to seek help too.

One thing is certain: if the family members get involved in family recovery of one kind or another, they are improving their own chances of happiness, and they are setting a tone of recovery in the household which will also improve chances for the addict. Whether the addict is ready or not, we strongly suggest that families seek help and enter the recovery process as soon as possible.

The sooner the family comes out in the open and lets the addict know they are seeking help for themselves, the sooner the "denial" of the problem will be penetrated. One approach is for family members to let the addict know they are receiving help, and give the addict an open invitation to participate as soon as he or she is ready.

Some family members seek help before there is any sign that the addict will stop; others do so because the recovering addict has suggested it. It is never too early to seek help, or to seek out an education about chemical dependency.

Doubts

Some family members resent having to seek help at all. They say to themselves:

> "Why do I need treatment? He's the one with the problem?"

> "I'm the one who's been doing everything around here. I don't need another thing to do!"

> "It's her problem. Let her work it out."

"I already know all this stuff—I don't need anyone's help."

"If he really loved me, he just wouldn't do it anymore!"

"What we really need is to just get all those dealers off the streets!"

"Why is she doing this to me?"

"I'm just going to leave her—I'm sure I can find a better wife."

"He promised me! This time I know it will be different!"

"I'm not like those people in those self-help groups."

"My situation is different."

"I can handle this on my own."

Most family members have had some of these thoughts at one time or another. The strain of living with someone with an addiction problem is enormous. It is hard to avoid feeling angry and sometimes wanting to blame the addict for everything.

Often, there is also a sense of shame associated with reaching out for help. If someone has been trying to handle the problem alone for a long time, it may seem like failure to finally seek help elsewhere. They might also fear others' reactions to the fact that someone in their life has a drug problem. The popular view of addicts may be that they are weak-willed, or "bad" people, but informed treatment professionals and members of support groups do not share this view. People in self-help groups are there because they've been through exactly the same thing themselves. They understand that it is an illness.

Family members will find that they no longer have to cope with this problem alone. Once they begin to educate themselves and get the support they need, their feelings of frustration and helplessness are often relieved.

Whether the addict is one's spouse, parent, child, sibling, friend, work associate, girlfriend or boyfriend there is help available to make it easier to deal with the addict, and one's own feelings.

UNANTICIPATED "LOSSES" IN RECOVERY

It is easy to think: "If the addict only stopped using cocaine, everything would be all right!"

Although this is what family members usually wish for, when it occurs, they may sometimes experience a different sort of problem. They've been accustomed to life being a certain way; to living in a constant state of crisis, or to focusing everything on the addict's problem. When the addict stops using and enters recovery, this can set off a series of changes in the family that can sometimes be uncomfortable.

For example, in a family with children, the addict may have had no part in disciplining the children for a long time. Having stopped using cocaine, he or she may now want to take an active role, one that may possibly conflict with that of the other parent. The parent who has born the brunt of the responsibility up until this point may resent the addict's sudden intrusion.

These conflicts are normal, and in time can be worked through. What are some of the other changes, or "losses," family members experience?

Glamorous Lifestyle

The addict may have accustomed the family to extravagant gifts/vacations/nights out as a result of the money earned through dealing cocaine. He or she may have treated the family members to parties or social events which he or she no longer wants to attend for fear of succumbing to temptation.

Feelings of Superiority Over the Addict

Family members may have grown accustomed to the addict's incompetence or irresponsibility. When the addict stops using, he or she may take back his or her own responsibilities, and this can sometimes be hard for family members to accept. Feelings of superiority and inferiority often occur in recovering families.

Drama of Constant Crises or Addict's Mood Swings

The family may have become accustomed to dealing with crises, or the addict's mood swings between getting "high" and "crashing" from cocaine. Paradoxically, life may feel dull when these mood swings even out. Sometimes family members may even miss the addict's "highs" and the accompanying excitement. Furthermore, the addict may experience depression in early recovery, which can also be hard for family members to deal with.

Feeling of Being Needed

Social isolation is a common symptom of cocaine addiction. Often the addict will rely heavily on family members for emotional support and company, just as the other family members come to rely on each other. As the addict and other family members recover, they will all enlarge their circles of support. This may mean that some of the family members may feel neglected, possibly even abandoned. They were needed before, but now they may feel unappreciated and undervalued. It is important for all family members to make the recovery transition at roughly the same pace and develop support resources of their own outside the immediate family itself.

Familiar Roles in the Family

When dealing with an addiction, the members of most addict's families adjust their roles in some way to cope. When the addict stops using cocaine, roles often need adjustment again, and this may be uncomfortable. If a father has a cocaine problem, his son may have become the "man about the house." The father in recovery may vehemently want to take back his parental and spousal role; friction with his son results. Both will need more flexibility than they are accustomed to.

"Victim" or "Martyr" Role

As discussed in the section on "co-dependency" and "enabling," family members may often find themselves sacrificing their own well-being in trying to help the addict. This creates an underlying resentment that often results in the family member feeling like a "victim," or "martyr."

In family self-help groups, one often hears the statement "There are no victims — there are only volunteers." This means that much of the suffering that a loved one's cocaine addiction causes, has been invited by the covert collaboration with the addiction itself. Breaking from this collaboration, and these harmful roles, requires positive action and a willingness to view familiar circumstances in a new way. This is not easy.

These ideas may seem paradoxical. But people do often adapt to harm in ways that themselves turn out to be harmful. These pitfalls need to be identified and accepted if the family is going to fully recover. Seeking counseling and taking part in self-help groups are ways of accomplishing this.

FAMILY RECOVERY

What a family can expect from recovery depends on factors such as: the help available to them, their commitment to working on their *own* recovery, their own inner strengths and resources, and whether the situation of the addict improves. There is no guarantee that because the family enters recovery, the addict will. Some families must decide whether they want to stay with the addict if he or she will not get help. This decision can be excruciating, and a family that has been pushed to this point should examine the choice from all angles.

Families that *do* survive entering recovery together can experience renewed family bonds and mutual love and supportiveness. Some families view their struggle with the addiction problem as a source of strength that enhances their lives more than they had imagined possible.

If family members make the difficult commitment to work on their own recovery — regardless of the addict's progress — their lives *will* improve. They will have gained new tools to handle anxiety, fear, disappointment, anger, depression, frustration and helplessness. They will see that they can be firm without being punitive and can say no without feeling guilty. They will no longer be dominated by people, problems or situations, and will learn how to enjoy life without waiting for "the axe to fall," or "the other shoe to drop." All this can mean new courage, peace of mind, self-confidence, emotional/spiritual development and love. This may sound too good to be true, but it is not. We have the families to prove it!

Unfortunately, some family members don't make this commitment to themselves. If the addict stops getting help, they do too. In most cases, they have failed to understand the need for their own recovery. They are still thinking about the addict's problems, not their own.

Indeed, it is enormously difficult to change old patterns of behavior. Families by their very nature are emotionally entwined and cannot be objective. While insight and intellectual understanding of the problems of addiction are helpful, insight into oneself is more important. And the key is positive action, the determination to break through old fears and compromises. Finally, the most important thing is to begin.

TREATMENT OPTIONS

Outpatient Psychotherapy/Counseling

Family members can choose to seek counseling from a professional. The following are suitable questions for determining the professional's experience in family work with addiction/alcoholism:

- **Do you work with families or individuals?**
  Often professionals treat both, but some focus mainly on individuals. If you want your whole family involved, you will need someone experienced in family therapy.
- **To what extent have you worked with alcoholism and addiction?**
  You want the professional to have worked with several clients who are alcoholic/addicts, and with their families.
- **What specific training do you have in alcoholism/addiction?**
  Some professionals take specific seminars/symposiums on chemical dependency. Others are specialists — e.g., "Certified

Alcoholism Counselors.'' Not all psychiatrists, psychologists or social workers are knowledgeable about addiction — many of them need additional training in addictive disorders and their treatment.

— **What supervised experience have you had in treating families with addiction problems?**
Their response to this question will probably give you an idea of how extensive their experience with families really is.

— **What self-help organizations are you familiar with?**
Listen for Alcoholics Anonymous, Al-Anon Family Groups, Cocaine Anonymous, Co-Anon Family Groups, Narcotics Anonymous, Nar-Anon, Families Anonymous, Co-dependents Anonymous.

— **Have you attended any of their meetings?**
To have an adequate understanding, it is helpful for professionals to attend some meetings.

— **Are you affiliated with any alcoholism treatment centers/ organizations?**
Some professionals work in alcoholism/addiction rehabilitation centers, or are members of organizations such as the local Alcoholism Council.

— **Do you think it's okay for a cocaine addict who stops using cocaine to drink alcohol?**
Some professionals believe recovering addicts can drink alcohol, others see alcohol as a drug and recommend total abstinence from any such mind-altering substance. As mentioned earlier, we think alcohol is dangerous for the recovering cocaine addict.

Psychotherapeutic counseling can consist of:

— Individual therapy (therapist and patient)
— Group therapy (therapist(s) and several patients)
— Family therapy (therapist(s), and family members, with or without the addict)
— Multiple-family therapy (therapist(s) and more than one family together)

Some of the goals of psychotherapeutic treatment are:

— Finding solutions to the problems that initially brought you to treatment
— Learning to see the choices you have in any situation
— Recognizing and understanding your feelings
— Developing your own strengths
— Improving self-esteem
— Improving communication skills and quality of relationships

Residential Treatment

Some addicts go to treatment centers where they live for several days or weeks and receive an intensive course consisting of psycho-therapy, educational seminars, group meetings and exposure to self-help groups. These facilities range from "detoxification centers" (where the addict stays until serious medical complications from withdrawal have subsided), to "inpatient" programs (consisting of varying degrees of therapy, educational seminars, group sessions and self-help meetings), to "therapeutic communities" (where the addict lives for a longer period of time until he or she is ready to rejoin society at large), to "halfway houses" (shared accommodation with other addicts as a "bridge" back to the community).

Some treatment centers want family members to participate in treatment, others do not. Some will not work with an addict unless the family agrees to take part; and others will invite the family for optional evening seminars/groups or provide "family week," where the family spends three days to an entire week at the center. Many facilities also introduce family members to family self-help programs. We have found that some degree of family participation in the addict's treatment is generally helpful, if the situation permits.

If the cocaine addict or family members decide they want help, one way to start looking is to call local hospitals or mental health centers. Referrals to private practitioners through friends can also be a good source.

There are a number of self-help groups which can be helpful for families and friends of cocaine addicts. We recommend the following:

- Co-Anon Family Groups
  (For families and friends of people abusing cocaine and other drugs)
- Nar-Anon
  (For families and friends of people abusing narcotics)
- Families Anonymous
  (For parents and other family members of people abusing cocaine and other drugs)
- Al-Anon Family Groups
  (For families and friends of alcoholics)

Co-Anon and Nar-Anon are specifically designed to help families concerned with drug addiction. If they do not exist in your area, Al-Anon offers the same wisdom and support from the perspective of families dealing with alcoholism. Although families of cocaine addicts are dealing with some specific problems particular to cocaine, the model of Al-Anon is the basis of all other Twelve-Step family self-help groups, and is therefore highly applicable and useful when dealing with cocaine-related family problems.

It is often found helpful for family members to sit in on Cocaine Anonymous meetings. Firsthand knowledge about addiction can be gained through listening to recovering cocaine addicts talk about their addiction — and subsequent recovery.

Family self-help programs provide literature on addiction and the family member's part in the problem. Group members meet regularly to discuss how they cope with the addiction of a friend or loved one. Their "recovery program" is based on the twelve steps of Alcoholics Anonymous (adapted for their own use), and their chief aim is for family members to regain a healthy level of functioning which is as healthy as possible, whether the addict is still using or not.

Chapter 9

Questions and Answers

What is freebase cocaine?

Freebase is a form of cocaine which is smoked. Cocaine becomes freebase through a chemical process of mixing baking soda or ether with water, and then with cocaine hydrochloride. A powerful "rush" is smoking's usual result, with the drug's effects being felt within two to three seconds, faster than through snorting or injection. Freebase cocaine is usually smoked in a water pipe to cool the harshness of the smoke.

What is crack?

Crack is simply freebase cocaine that is packaged and sold in small vials, smaller than those for perfume samples. Each of these usually holds three or four nuggets resembling white pebbles. The price ranges from $2 to $25 depending on the cocaine's quality and the part of the country in which it is sold. It's name comes from the crackling sound it makes when smoked. Crack is a convenient way to use cocaine because it is pre-packaged and ready to smoke.

What is a "crack house"?

A crack house is a place where a person can buy and smoke crack. Crack houses are also called "base" or "rock" houses. Abandoned buildings in low income neighborhoods are often used.

What is an "8-ball"?

An 8-Ball is a slang term used to designate 1/8th of an ounce of cocaine, approximately 4 grams. Users might say "We did an 8-ball."

What are "cocaine bugs"?

Cocaine users have reported feeling imagined bugs or insects on their bodies while under the influence of cocaine. Some reported scratching themselves until they had sores.

What is a "speed ball"?

A speed ball is a mixture of cocaine and heroin; it can be either snorted or injected. The two drugs are mixed in order to combine the stimulant effect of the cocaine and the depressant effect of the heroin.

What is basuco?

Basuco is a paste that is derived from coca leaves, and is usually mixed with marijuana or tobacco and then smoked. Central and South Americans smoke basuco because it is less expensive than other forms of cocaine. The paste is considered unclean since it contains lead and petroleum by-products created by the process for extracting cocaine from the leaves.

What is a "rush"?

A rush is the initial, intense feeling caused by the intake of cocaine.

What is the "crash?"

The crash occurs after the initial effects of cocaine have worn off. It is experienced as a severe letdown, similar to depression. This letdown feeling is both psychological and physical.

How can an employer tell if an employee is using cocaine?

Serious cocaine users will show the effects of their use at work. They will exhibit several of the following symptoms.

- lateness or absences
- frequent trips to the bathroom
- weight loss
- irritability and outbursts of anger
- mood swings

- increased number of personal telephone calls
- secretiveness
- associating with suspected drug users
- change in personal hygiene
- change in attitude
- stealing from the job or asking for unreasonable advances

Is crack a poor man's drug?

Since crack is initially inexpensive, crack dealers market the drug to the poorer people. Crack use is not only destroying poor people as individuals but it is destroying their communities. Drug dealers have taken possession of abandoned buildings, usually located in low-income neighborhoods, and frighten residents into passive acceptance of their drug selling. However, crack dealers are more frightening because of their influence on the young people in the ghetto. The dealers work openly, too often becoming role models because of their fast rise to money and prestige. Adolescents are usually first introduced to crack when they become couriers taking crack from the dealer to the seller. They are used as couriers because they cannot be prosecuted as adults if they are convicted of selling the drug. Some seek the job solely for the money, but most soon become addicted to the drug.

Can crack be smoked in a regular pipe?

Crack can be smoked in anything, even a soda can that will hold the pellet and enables the smoker to inhale the drug through the mouth. However, there are specialized pipes of clear glass in which water is placed to cool the smoke before it enters the lungs. Since crack comes in ready-to-smoke pellets, all that is necessary is an instrument to hold the pellet and a match or lighter to light it.

What does it feel like to be high on cocaine?

Most people report euphoria, a sense of well-being; this includes the conviction that they are in total control. That euphoric experience doesn't last, and a user soon becomes trapped in the effort to recreate it.

Is cocaine easy to buy?

It depends upon where one lives, works and plays. It is easier to obtain in cities and large towns, although it can be found in small, midwestern towns as well. Cocaine is very accessible in low-income, urban areas and cosmopolitan suburbs. Many people are able to buy cocaine where they work, whether it be Wall Street or a small construction company. Students can easily buy cocaine in school.

Can cocaine be used without causing addiction?

We don't think so, and more importantly, the risk isn't worth it. Treatment centers and jails are full of people who began by using cocaine socially. There is no way that anyone can determine who can use cocaine and not become addicted. So why take the chance?

Is there a safe way to use cocaine?

No, cocaine is addicting in any form. While smoking and injecting cocaine seems to cause addiction more quickly than snorting it, people who snort cocaine become just as addicted.

Is there a cure for cocaine addiction?

The only cure that works 100% of the time is abstinence from cocaine and other drugs, including alcohol. At the very least, it is necessary to abstain from cocaine use. We have seen people begin using cocaine again after drinking alcohol or smoking marijuana. Taking a drug lowers one's inhibitions, including those against drug use. Drinking can also sharpen the craving itself, whetting the users' appetite.

Is cocaine dangerous for pregnant women?

While cocaine use is dangerous for everyone, its effects can be devastating on an unborn child. Cocaine is absorbed directly by the fetus through the amniotic sac. There is no protection from the drug.

What about nursing mothers, can they use cocaine?

Absolutely not, because, as with pregnant women, the cocaine is directly absorbed by the baby.

Does cocaine enhance sexual desire?

Many cocaine addicts say that at first cocaine enhanced sexual desire. After prolonged use however, they found sex became unimportant and their sexual activity dwindled. Only the drug mattered.

I don't use cocaine but someone I live with keeps it in our home. Can I get in trouble from this?

If cocaine is found on the premises by police with a search warrant you will be suspected of possession unless the other person confesses to ownership.

What should I do if I find cocaine paraphernalia in my child's room?

This is not something to be taken lightly. Consider calling your local drug abuse agency and asking for help. Let the experts help you help your child.

Is there cocaine withdrawal?

There is a withdrawal known as the cocaine crash. The depression and craving, however, do not constitute a withdrawal similar to that faced by an alcoholic or a user of tranquilizers or heroin. These people are usually detoxified with decreasing amounts of sedatives to ease the withdrawal symptoms, which include nausea, headaches and vomiting. Cocaine addicts are not usually detoxified with sedatives.

How can someone be addicted to cocaine if that person only uses once a month?

The question of addiction does not depend on the amount and frequency of cocaine use. One can be addicted to cocaine if he or she uses it once every four months. If cocaine use disrupts the person's life in any way—financially, emotionally or physically—it probably signals a problem. If you think that you may use cocaine too much, the chances are that you do.

What is a cocaine relapse?

A cocaine relapse is when someone uses cocaine after a period of abstinence.

Are cocaine addicts more susceptible to AIDS?

Yes, in two ways: (1) in sharing needles with other addicts (a cocaine addict who injects cocaine); (2) they are more likely to be exposed to the the virus through sexual promiscuity which is common in cocaine addicts. Many cocaine addicts have reported that part of the cocaine addiction involved sexual promiscuity. Many women admit that they prostituted themselves for cocaine. Many men and women said they enjoyed sex more under cocaine's influence, and therefore were very sexually active.

Is drug testing helpful for cocaine addicts in treatment centers?

Drug testing is often an effective treatment technique in which the addict's urine is tested for the chemical traces of cocaine or other drugs. Many addicts appreciate the testing as a deterrent to drug use. It is helpful to establish the facts with such tests. Many addicts lie about their drug use; the tests expose their falsehoods. Others may not use drugs, but appear to be. In their cases, testing clears them of suspicion.

How can I turn down an offer of cocaine and not look square or stupid?

This is a crucial question for a recovering addict, especially adolescents concerned about what their peers think. The fear of looking square or stupid is one of the leading causes of relapse and a common reason people give when asked why they used cocaine in the first place. It is crucial that you do not give in to the mistaken idea that you look good by using cocaine. When you feel good about yourself, you do not have to take a drug to prove that you are "cool" or "okay." Using cocaine to look good means running the risk of addiction to please others.

If I stop using cocaine, won't my life become boring?

If you work at building a new lifestyle, you will not be bored. By participating in some form of treatment program you will meet other people, like yourself, who are trying to stop using cocaine. They are discovering how to enjoy life and involvement with them can be exhilarating. The most beneficial step, however, may be to think about the activities you once enjoyed, before cocaine took over your life, and then do *something!*

Is sex going to be different without cocaine?

Some former cocaine users have reported that they are now more inhibited and find it difficult to perform as they once did. Many others feel, however, that sex is more fulfilling and there is a deeper enjoyment when drugs are not involved.

What should a person do when they get an urge to use cocaine?

When a person gets a drug craving, he or she must think through the drug craving. They need to think about the beginning of using the drug and follow it through to the end: crashing from cocaine; out of money, and with their loved ones' knowledge that they have used cocaine. It is wise to remember that using cocaine will worsen any situation. It is also useful to call someone who is supportive of staying clean.

What should I do if I have a relapse?

Don't give up because you think you have failed. Many people have recovered after having had a relapse. It's important to find someone who will be understanding and supportive. Do not get high again. Get involved with your support people.

What should a person do if they've stopped using cocaine and their life doesn't seem to improve?

Have patience. Most cocaine addicts want results immediately. They look for instant gratification: this is part of drug addiction, especially cocaine addiction. Cocaine gets a person high almost immediately. The cocaine addict wants to experience sobriety the way he or she experienced cocaine, almost instantly.

The passage of time is required before a life begins to mend. The impatient person needs to look at others who are doing well and try to understand that if they can stay straight they will be just as successful.

What does recovering and recovery mean?

"Recovering" is a term used by addicts who are participating in a Twelve-Step program. It means that an addict cannot be cured of the disease. There is always a possibility of being actively addicted again. Recovery is the process of learning to how to live life without using any drug, including alcohol.

What is a Twelve-Step program?

The first Twelve-Step program was created in 1935 by two alcoholics who formed Alcoholics Anonymous. There are now numerous Twelve-Step programs, including Cocaine Anonymous, Co-Anon, Narcotics Anonymous, Nar-Anon, Al-Anon, Drugs Anonymous, Adult Children of Alcoholics (ACOA), Overeaters Anonymous, Sexaholics Anonymous, Gamblers Anonymous, Debtors Anonymous, Gamanon, Emotions Anonymous and Families Anonymous. Each program has a unique emphasis, but all are based on the principles of the twelve steps and twelve traditions of Alcoholics Anonymous. The twelve steps are outlined in the Prologue. It should be recognized that while the language reflects the 1930s, the concepts are flexible and open to all kinds of interpretations.

What do the words sober, clean and dry mean?

Sober, clean and dry mean that the person is abstaining from all drugs, including alcohol. There are differences in that a "sober" or "clean" person is alcohol- and drug-free, and participates in a Twelve-Step program. A "dry" person abstains from drugs and alcohol but not with the help of a Twelve-Step recovery program.

Can a former drug addict take prescribed drugs?

Yes, if he or she is honest with the doctor about the history of drug abuse. Many doctors are not familiar with addiction and it is the recovering addict's responsibility to ensure that the medications are safe and nonaddictive. If it is necessary to take addictive drugs, then it is crucial that the doses are monitored. It can be dangerous because addicts have been known to relapse after taking prescribed drugs.

What are some common terms for drugs?

Heroin is sometimes called smack, horse, doogi, dope, white lady, brown sugar, scag or salt and pepper. Marijuana is sometimes called pot, reefer, grass, Mary Jane, weed or dope. Amphetamines are called ups, dex, meth, white lightening, beauties, white crosses, uppers, speed, crank, or ice.

Chapter 10

A New Life:
Conclusion

What is life like after one has stopped using cocaine? Here is what a group of recovering cocaine addicts and their families have to say about their new lives.

"What's my life like today since I am not using coke?" John asked aloud as he looked down at his folded hands in his lap. After a minute or two, he sighed, looked up and a bright smile lit his face.

> I have a life today. I didn't have one before. I lived for cocaine. I lived for no one or nothing else, not even me. I had no real relationships with people, including myself. I didn't know who I was, and truthfully, I didn't really care. All that mattered to me was "doing up some coke." My family, my job, my health, everything was secondary to getting high on cocaine. The sad thing about it is that I never knew that this was happening while I was in the middle of my addiction. I guess that is what denial is. It sure works. It worked for me because I did not believe it was the cocaine that was creating the problems in my life.
>
> I thought that I was in "control," never realizing that the cocaine was really in "control." Today I can see clearly that I was going nowhere, I didn't like myself. I didn't care about others. Physically, I was a wreck. What more can I say except that at the time I thought this was life!
>
> Today I can't say enough about how good I feel about myself, that I do care about others especially my family and

friends. I have a future that is positive, and my body works. In fact, this is the first time in my life that I feel healthy. Most important, I have hope today. The word hope was not in my vocabulary while I used cocaine. I believe that you cannot have hope when cocaine rules your life.

John stopped, swallowed hard and wiped his moist eyes, a little self-consciously. He looked at his wife Meghan who was sitting by his side openly crying. Meghan sniffled and she began to talk:

I can't believe how much our lives have changed. John is right; we had no relationship. While I hoped and hoped that he would stop using cocaine, deep down I wasn't sure if he could stop. We had no life together. Now I can sleep through the night without worrying about where he is. I don't have to check the bank balance every day to make sure that he didn't spend all our money. My God, I don't know how I lived like that. Don't get me wrong, we still have our fights but at least he is here to fight with. That is what is so amazing, that John is here and I am here, and we are together.

Not only are couples brought together but all kinds of relationships can be healed when the addict stops using cocaine and obtains help.

"If I had known what life would be like without cocaine, I would have stopped using a long time ago," said Lauren fiercely. "Especially since I spent precious years with cocaine rather than with my daughter. Those years are gone, and I cannot wish them back, no matter how hard I try. I cannot redo the past."

Lauren reached over and put her arm around her twelve-year-old daughter Katherine's shoulders. Katherine reached up and squeezed her mother's hand. It was obvious that both mother and daughter shared a strong and genuine affection. Lauren went on:

"Do you realize that I never used to touch my daughter? When I tried, she would back away from me like I was some sort of monster. I guess I was in some ways.''

> It is unbelievable that life holds such possibilities for me, possibilities that I never knew existed. You see, in the midst of my cocaine addiction, I didn't know there was another and better way to live. When I used coke, I felt so guilty but I didn't know how to relieve the guilt except to use more cocaine! I was so ashamed when I went home at five in the morning and Katherine would be waiting up for me. She was crying and wondering where I had been. I felt worthless when my family turned away in disgust when I asked for money to pay my cocaine debts. I was terrified to look at the bills because I had spent the money on cocaine. My daughter had no clothes for special occasions; cocaine was more important. I dreaded waking up in the morning to face a new day without cocaine when my supply was gone.
> Today I have none of this. I love to wake up in the morning because I know that I did not use cocaine the night before. My daughter still cries but I am there for her when she does. I can't say enough for being in the real world, not a cocaine-induced one. Yes, life has its ups and downs, and recovery from cocaine addiction is not easy. I wouldn't trade my recovery for the world.

Lauren looked at Katherine and asked, "What do you think? Do you think our relationship is better now?" Katherine shyly responded by whispering:

> It's better than before. I was ashamed of my mother. I couldn't bring my friends home because I didn't know if she would be high on cocaine or crashing from it. My friends knew that she was into crack and felt sorry for me. I just wanted to hide in my room. My dad was never there so I had only my mother and she wasn't there. She never helped me with my homework. She didn't notice whether or not I went to school. She never came to the parent functions, which made me feel unloved and different from all the other kids. I have to admit that

watching her recover from addiction has been tough. We still have fights, and now I have to come home by a certain time when before I could stay out all night. I have had to change too because now I can't blame my mother for all my problems. It was easy to blame her. I could always make excuses for my poor grades or lack of friends; now I can't do that. Even though this makes it tougher in some ways, I have never once, no matter how mad I've been at my mother, wished that she would go away and do crack. I couldn't take it anymore. I used to wish that I had a different mother. You know, today I don't wish that. I am glad she is my mother.

After a minute or two, a clear voice rang out saying, "You people are lucky because you have people like your parents or wife. The one person I really cared about died a few years ago and I feel so bad that he never saw me straight." The voice belonged to Bobby, a wiry young man, who gestured eloquently with his hands. Bobby threw his hands up and cried,

I always hated my father. He beat me, you know, to show me that "he was the boss," and I swore I would get even. Well I sure did because as soon as I could I started staying out late at night running with the guys and coming home stoned on crack. By then I could hit him back so he wouldn't touch me. I look back on that today and realize that even though he had no right to hit me or treat me the way he did, he did the best he could. After all, he was an alcoholic who came from a home where his father beat him. Anyway, I wish he could see that I'm straight today and trying to do the right thing.

I also see that the person I was really hurting was me. It was my life that I was destroying. Well, no more, I'm not destroying my life. Now I have to learn a new way to live. I am learning how to think, talk and be different from the old Bobby who used to rip people off and get fired from job after job. It's hard because I sure do have a temper. I have to keep it in check, but it's worth it. I listen to you people and all my new friends who are trying to stay off the coke and I believe I have a chance. I didn't have a chance before. Now I do, and I don't want to blow it. Someday I will relate to a woman and all that stuff. Right now I have to focus on Bobby and get well. I must recover from this addiction that almost took my life.

Everyone in the group clapped, saying, "Way to go, Bobby." Bobby grinned self-consciously. "And one more thing," Bobby said, "If anyone every clapped for me when I was using coke, I would punch that sucker as hard as I could because I figured everyone was out to get me or make fun of me."

"I'm a father and maybe I can help you, Bobby, with my story," said Pete. Pete, a burly, barrel-chested man, looks around the room before sharing what life was like when his son was getting high and how much better life is today.

My son, Jim, has always been strong-willed and independent. When he started using cocaine, however, he became impossible. My wife, Roseann and I, never knew if he was telling the truth. We had to start hiding our money and jewelry because we found it missing on occasion. The worst was when we discovered he had stolen one of our checks from our checkbook and forged my signature to get money to buy cocaine.

Jim was skipping school and his grades went down. He was looking worse physically and had a terrible attitude. It was as if we had become the enemy. He refused to talk to us. We had lost total authority over him. Finally, he hit his bottom and got help. At first, this was difficult because we didn't know how to act, whether we should be his friends or parents. Slowly, we started to adjust to the change and were able to help in the right ways.

It has been such a relief not waiting at night wondering if he will make it home, we are also able to keep our money and jewelry in our home. Building up the trust between us has taken time and has not come easy. There are still times when Jim is late, or doesn't tell us where he's going. Then we think that he is getting high again. We talk to each other and help each other through these times. We also call other people who have had similar experiences as ours. They are more objective and help us keep the focus on ourselves, and not worry about Jim.

Jim has become the teenager we knew and loved before he got into cocaine. I'm not saying that he is a saint, remember he is a teenager! All in all, however, there is no comparison to what he was like while he used cocaine and now. For that, we are very grateful.

Everyone's eyes turned to Jim, a lanky teenager with a touch of acne. Jim was the only one in the group who had not spoken and he did not appear very eager to begin. After a minute of uncomfortable silence for Jim, he cleared his throat.

"Well, I am probably not the easiest guy to live with," he admitted with a frown. "I don't have much of a sense of humor. I also know that I am a little sensitive to what I think is criticism."

"Which is asking him to do anything around the house," said Pete, with a smile. Jim gave a small smile in return and sighed.

Well, dad, it's not easy being a teenager. All the kids think I'm a nerd now that I don't use coke or any drugs or alcohol. It is also hard to talk to girls without anything in me to give me courage. Oh, listen to me. Boy, do I feel sorry for me. Yeah, it's difficult, but I know that this is better than when I was depressed during the crashes from coke. I have to remember that the kids who give me a hard time about not using drugs are the ones who have a problem with drugs.

My mother is okay too, and she is trying really hard. She tries not to do everything for me like she used to. She is trying to let me grow up. So we are all changing, and for the better. We talk today and we try to listen to each other. I never used to listen to anybody and I sure didn't think anyone ever listened to me. So my world is a different and better one. I didn't have a world when I used cocaine and other drugs. I had a miserable existence, one that I don't want again. I'm actually lucky! Because I'm so young, I meet a lot of older people who have a lot of regrets about having spent most of their lives on drugs. I don't have to do that and I sure don't want to.

The group was silent, but the silence was comfortable. It was amazing that this group of very different people felt so obviously at home with each other.

On the other hand, maybe it was not so amazing. After all, at one time everyone had been in the same place. Now, each is traveling on the same journey—toward a drug-free life. It is a journey that they all agree is worth its destination: a happy, joyous and free life.

Chapter 11

Where to Get Help
and Find Treatment Resources

TWELVE-STEP PROGRAM RESOURCES

Cocaine Anonymous

Cocaine Anonymous World Service Office
P.O. Box 1367
Culver City, California 90239
800-347-8998

Alcoholics Anonymous

Alcoholics Anonymous General Service Office
468 Park Avenue South
New York, New York 10016
Contact your local directory for phone number

Narcotics Anonymous

World Service Office Narcotics Anonymous
P.O. Box 9999
Van Nuys, California 91409
818-780-3951

Co-Anon

Co-Anon Family Groups
P.O. Box 64742-66
Los Angeles, California 90064
West of the Mississippi, call 213-859-2206
East of the Mississippi, call 212-713-5133

Al-Anon

Al-Anon Family Groups, Inc.
P.O. Box 862
Midtown Station
New York, New York 10018-0862
Contact your local telephone directory for the telephone number.

Nar-Anon

Nar-Anon Family Group Headquarters, Inc.
P.O. Box 2562
Palos Verdes Peninsula, California 90274
213-547-5800

OTHER RESOURCES

National Clearinghouse for Alcohol and Drug Information
P.O. Box 2345
Rockville, Maryland 20850
301-468-2600

National Council on Alcoholism, Inc.
12 West 21st Street
7th Floor
New York, New York 10010
212-206-6770

National Association for Children of Alcoholics
31706 Coast Highway
Suite 201
South Laguna, California 92677
714-499-3889

National Institute on Drug Abuse (N.I.D.A.)
Hotline 1-800-662-HELP

Index

Abstinence, as cocaine addiction treatment, 95,122
Acquired immune deficiency syndrome (AIDS), 124
Adolescents
  cocaine addiction, 49-60
    bingeing, 54
    case examples, 49-52
    effects, 52-55
    factors affecting, 52-53
    interventions, 56-59
    misperceptions regarding, 52-53
    parental responses, 55-59,77-82
    questionnaire, 61
    school's preventive role, 59-60
    signs of, 55-56
  crack use, 6,121
AIDS. *SEE* Acquired immune deficiency syndrome
Al-Anon, 2,118,138
Alcoholics Anonymous (A.A.), 126,137
  adolescents' participation, 58,60
  twelve-steps, 2-3. *See also* Twelve-Step programs
Alcoholism, development of, 14
Alcohol use, cocaine use correlation, 54-55,67-69,71,95,122
Amphetamines
  as cocaine adulterants, 11
  common names, 127
Anesthetics, as cocaine adulterants, 11,12

Basuco, 14,120
Bias, Len, 6
"Bingeing", 7,8,15,54
Boundary setting, by cocaine addict's family, 98-99,107-108
Brain, cocaine's effects on, 8-9,11

Bromocriptine, 8,14

Caffeine, as cocaine adulterant, 11
Cardiovascular system, cocaine's effects on, 6-7,10,12-13
Children, of cocaine addicts, 96,97
Co-Anon, 2,137
Coca-Cola, 5
Cocaine
  administration routes, 10-14
    addiction risk correlation, 122
    intranasal inhalation, 10-11,17
    intravenous injection, 11-12,17,124
    smoking, 12-14,17
  adulterants, 11,12
  anesthetic effects, 5,6,10
  behavioral effects, 18
  biochemical effects, 6-9
  as illegal substance, 95-96,123
  misperceptions regarding, 52-54
  origin, 5-6
  physical effects, 17-18
    physiological effects, 7-10,11,12-13
  psychological effects, 18
  purchase of, 122
  sexual effects, 9-10,15,123,124,125
  "speedballs", 11,20
  stimulant effects, 5,6-9
  withdrawal, 8,14,120,123
Cocaine addiction
  administration route correlation, 12
  alcohol use correlation, 54-55,67-69,71, 95,122
  "bingeing", 7,8,15,54
  case examples, 21-46
  criminal activity and, 54,95-96,123
  cure, 122
  development time, 14

Milton Keynes UK
Ingram Content Group UK Ltd.
UKHW040712141024
449569UK00005B/112